D1526004

Classics in Psychiatry

A

PRACTICAL ACCOUNT

OF

GENERAL PARALYSIS

Th[omas] J. Austin

ARNO PRESS

A New York Times Company

New York • 1976

Editorial Supervision: EVE NELSON

———◆———

Reprint Edition 1976 by Arno Press Inc.

Reprinted from a copy in
  The Duke University Library

CLASSICS IN PSYCHIATRY
ISBN for complete set: 0-405-07410-7
See last pages of this volume for titles.

Manufactured in the United States of America

———◆———

Library of Congress Cataloging in Publication Data

Austin, Thomas J
  A practical account of general paralysis.

  (Classics in psychiatry)
  Reprint of the 1859 ed. published by J. Churchill,
London.
  1. Neurosyphylis. I. Title. II. Series.
[DNLM: WL A938p 185a]
RC201.7.N4A9 1975   616.8'92   75-16681
ISBN 0-405-07413-1

A

PRACTICAL ACCOUNT

OF

GENERAL PARALYSIS,

ITS

MENTAL AND PHYSICAL SYMPTOMS, STATISTICS,

CAUSES, SEAT, AND TREATMENT.

BY

THOS. J. AUSTIN, M.R.C.S., ENG.

LATELY MEDICAL OFFICER AT BETHNAL HOUSE ASYLUM.

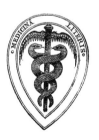

LONDON:

JOHN CHURCHILL, NEW BURLINGTON STREET.

MDCCCLIX.

PRINTED BY J. E. ADLARD,
BARTHOLOMEW CLOSE, E.C.

ADVERTISEMENT.

THE short account of General Paralysis contained in the following pages, is principally based on the author's personal experience. While medical officer at Bethnal House Asylum, and subsequently, a large number of general paralytics have come under his notice. From the study, and from the histories of these cases, and from the collation of their post-mortem appearances, he has drawn, with however unskilful a hand, the portrait, ascertained the causes, and fixed, as he believes, the seat of the disease.

To the late Mr. Phillips he is indebted for an introduction to the subject, and for whatever reliable information he has been able to gather regarding the first stage of the malady.

5, RIVER STREET, MYDDELTON SQUARE;
December, 1858.

CONTENTS.

CHAPTER II.

CHAPTER III.

CHAPTER IV.

CHAPTER VII.

GENERAL PARALYSIS.

INTRODUCTION.

GENERAL paralysis, though it had doubtless existed from the earliest period of insanity, eluded observation, or at least never so fixed the attention of those who must have witnessed it, as to be recognised and described as a distinct disease, till the early part of the present century.

Though since the date of its discovery it has been known to the superintendents of lunatic asylums, and to those medical men who have devoted themselves to the study of insanity, it has been practically unknown to the body of the profession, and by many of its members it has never been heard of.

This want of knowledge is easily accounted for : it is indeed precisely what was to be expected of a disease which was not mentioned by medical lecturers, or described by the authors of class-books—which was not seen, or at least not recognised in general hospitals.

No separate volume on the subject has, as far as I know, been published by a British author, though it has been incidentally mentioned, or imperfectly described, by writers and lecturers on insanity. To supply the want is the intention of the present work. Though intended principally for the perusal of those who have *not* made an especial study of insanity, it may possibly contain some facts and views not unworthy the attention of professed psychologists.

Beside the comparative novelty of the subject, and the absence of any book on it, its intrinsic importance demands the publicity of whatever may be known regarding it. And here let me premise that it is a perfectly distinct disease from ordinary paralysis—the result of cerebro-spinal compression or disorganization—distinct in its symptoms and treatment, in its epoch, causes, and seat. It is important that the disease should be well known, because it is not uncommon, and is said to be increasing disproportionably to the increase of population. Whether this increase is real, may be perhaps doubted; at least it is still an open question. The more easy recognition of the malady has possibly produced the apparent increase; though, on the other hand, it is equally likely that the wear and tear of modern society, the intense and therefore frequently unsuccessful struggle for position or livelihood, which is everywhere going on around us, and which is so characteristic of our age, and the more frequent occurrence of mental anguish, the consequence of domestic trials, may have actually augmented the number of its victims. It is important the disease should be better known than heretofore, because it is to be feared that, even among the superintendents of asylums, sufficient attention has not been paid to the subject after the recognition of the disease, from the assumption, unhappily but too well founded, of its incurability; while the general want of knowledge regarding the diagnostic symptoms of its early and, if ever, curable stage, has hitherto deprived the patient of all chance of mending his condition.

Irrespective of its purely medical point of view, the early recognition of the malady is a matter of importance legally, and in respect of the happiness and welfare of individuals or families. That mental aberration, mere wandering of the mind, is an early psychical symptom of general paralysis, is very probable, but, if it be, the wandering is not permanent or great; the mind recovers itself, it regains the track whence it had deviated, and the energy remains sufficient to conceal the transient error from the world. As the disease advances, the controlling power diminishing and the aberration increasing, the mental unsoundness of its subject becomes evident. It is then only, and indeed not always then, that the physical disease is detected. The first overt act of insanity opens the eyes of the patient's family and medical attendant to his real condition: it is the climax of, and clue to, a long series of mental symptoms, which may, from their harmlessness, have passed by nearly unheeded; or, on the contrary, which may have been the cause of the greatest anguish or complete ruin to those who have been dependent on the incipient paralytic for advice or support; or which may have involved the patient himself in all manner of absurd or unfortunate predicaments. It is, therefore, highly desirable that the early physical symptoms of this malady should be ascertained and made known, so that the patient, while his mind is giving way, if he be still permitted to regulate his own actions, should at least be denied any control over the fate of others, which he may have heretofore enjoyed.

If, from the unobtrusive character of its primary physical symptoms, the detection of general paralysis is, in the present state of our knowledge, difficult or impossible in its earliest stage, it is alike possible and easy to detect it in its matured or second stage. Its recognition at this period is the more important, as its subject, however much his mental and physical condition may be improved, is henceforth (as far as my experience goes) unfitted to resume his place in the social system; he is no longer capable of rightly directing his energies for his own benefit, and still less of conducting that nice mental and moral operation which directs them for the benefit of others.

CHAPTER I.

MENTAL SYMPTOMS.

THE general plan I shall adopt in the treatment of the subject, will be first succinctly to describe the physical and, more fully, the mental symptoms of the disease; and then, as minutely as my knowledge permits me, to notice the condition of each external organ or tissue implicated, and the changes observable in such organs during the different stages of the malady.

For the convenience of description, the course of general paralysis may be divided into three stages; and I the more readily adopt this division, artificial though of course it be, as it is founded in reality. Each stage presents its distinct set of symptoms, mental and physical; the patient's condition is very different in each stage; and the prognosis, sometimes a matter of no mean importance, is entirely regulated by the period of the malady at which the paralytic has arrived. It is indeed true that the end of one stage imperceptibly merges into the commencement of the next; yet if the incipient symptoms of each stage be contrasted, the spectator might fairly suppose that not three phases of the same malady, but three distinct diseases, were before him.

The first stage of general paralysis extends from the commencement of the disease (a very uncertain date) to that epoch of it, when the insidiously advancing mental symptoms become so evident, as to convince the patient's friends of his madness, or at least to make them doubtful of his sanity ; so that the termination of this stage may be said to depend rather on the acumen of the patient's friends than on any symptom peculiar to this phase of his malady.

The second stage extends from the recognition of the actual or nascent insanity through an uncertain and greatly differing period of mental derangement, more or less complete, which is sometimes continuous and sometimes interrupted by lucid intervals, to a time when all the faculties of the mind give way, and more or less complete dementia begins.

The third and last stage extends from commencing dementia through a period of increasing mental and physical feebleness, which progresses, till the mind is a blank and the body scarce alive, to the inevitably fatal result.

Of the first, and by far the most interesting of the three stages, interesting alike from our ignorance of it and from its possible curability, little or next to nothing is known. To that little I cannot, from my own knowledge, add much. Nearly all that I have learned on the subject has been derived from the experience of the late Mr. Phillips; but the little light, which he was able to throw on it, is flickering and dim, for the opportunities of witnessing the stage were to him rare, and occurred to him accidentally. There being no marked mental symptoms, the patient does not come under the notice of those whose reputation is founded on their knowledge of insanity; and if his physical symptoms require medical interference, the real disease is not recognised, only because it has never been described, or, more truly, because its symptoms are unknown.

Nearly all the instances of this, the first stage of the malady, which were observed by Mr. Phillips, occurred in persons with whom he was accidentally brought in contact, and who at the time were supposed to be free from any paralytic, or, indeed, from any other affection. In these persons, all of whom became subsequently paralytic, he remarked a very singular circumstance— the contraction of the pupils to a point, and the complete and permanent destruction of their mobility, without, as far as he could ascertain, any diminution of visual power. As this phenomenon occurred principally in young blue or gray-eyed men, the appearance of the eyeball was very remarkable, from the mass ·of exposed light-coloured iris, unrelieved by the dark pupil. The next time Mr. Phillips saw any of these persons (and frequently months had elapsed before he saw them again) he observed a notable change in their manner and expression; they had become more vivacious, and seemed to overflow with animal spirits; they had a greater notion of their own importance or talents. Many sane men have as much vivacity and as great a self-complacency as these persons exhibited, coincident with their pin-point pupils; it was the change from their usual quiet demeanour which particularly struck him. After another long interval, he was again brought in contact with them. Their exuberance of spirits and self-satisfaction had increased. Then rumours shortly reached him of extravagancies or blunders having been committed in their respective vocations, which at length became so marked and numerous as seriously to interfere with the proper carrying on of their business. Hence arose expostulation on the part of those interested in their affairs; to no avail, however, for the incipient paralytic had now become irritable and headstrong, more than ever convinced of his own talents, and, in a word, completely impracticable. All this time the immediate friends did not perceive the immensity of the change which had taken place in him, and were unwilling to admit his incompetence to retain his commercial or professional position. Daily brought in contact with their relative or friend, they had become habituated to his increasing self-complacency and many eccentricities; and affection, even if it recognised the fact, took a lenient view of his failing memory and intellectual declension. Those, however, who saw him but seldom, having a point of departure in their previous meeting, recognised the change and commented on it. At length the psychical symptoms so increased, as to render his declining mental condition evident even to the dim eyes of friendship, and with more or less difficulty he was removed from his social position. Though arrived at this epoch of his disease, he could scarcely be said to have manifested any positive indications of insanity. The mental symptoms had been principally negative; impairment of memory and of the faculty of attention, a diminished consecutiveness in the ideas and actions, irritability and self-sufficiency, are not to be regarded as symptoms of an unsound, though they are doubtless those of a feeble, or of an ill-regulated, mind. In the incipient paralytic, however, exaggerated notion of mental power increases in an inverse ratio with real capacity; the less capable of healthy action the mind becomes, the more complete is the conviction of its competence for the performance of the most exalted intellectual achievements. These two operations — diminishing power and increasing estimate, going on *pari passu,* soon bring their subject to the verge of positive delusion—to such a state, that the law, always merciful to the insane, at length no longer hesitates to recognise him as *non compos mentis.* From an early period of his disease, indeed, he has been the victim of a gradually increasing delusion, an exaggerated estimate of his own powers. This, however, is so common a fancy in the otherwise sane, and so usually curable by the failures which result from it, that the interference of the law, or at least the protection of the lunacy statutes, is rarely invoked. But when the patient begins to have grand delusions, to fancy he is very rich, that he has large estates, a title or an immense family, his insanity is too evident for even the laws of England, how jealous soever of the liberty of the subject, not to acknowledge. It is at this date of his malady that he makes his appearance at the lunatic asylum, and is, according to my arrangement, at the commencement of the second stage.

Mr. Phillips noticed, that as the disease advances through its first stage, the contracted pupils enlarge, though rarely equally.

That the mental indications of the first stage are not always such as those observed by Mr. Phillips, is certain; for, at the commencement of the second stage, which is only the climax of the first, the symptoms are often very different from those I have just described.

The course of the subject now brings me to the consideration of the second stage of the disease; and I may here introduce a brief account of its physical signs.

Among the various diseases or derangements of the organism, of which the most marked symptom is insanity, there is not one which presents so striking or so consistent a group of physical signs as general paralysis. If a person who is insane, or who has shown gradually increasing mental declension, have slight tremors of the lips, especially of the upper lip; if the mouth be broad, straight, unchiselled, and devoid of its usual curves; if the pupils be irregular, unsymmetrical, or contracted and insensible; if the utterance be imperfect, or even so slightly affected as to show itself only in the jumbling of the syllables of some long word; if the facial aperture of the nostrils be of unequal size; if the mouth be opened unequally in the act of talking; if the tongue be large, flabby, and tremulous, protruded or not out of the mesian line; if the gait be feeble, straddling, or devious; the person in whom all these symptoms coincide, be his mental symptoms what they may, is the subject of general paralysis. That there are some cases of the disease in its second stage which do not present a concurrence of all these physical signs, is indeed true; thus, the pupils are not always unequal, the utterance is sometimes tolerably perfect, the gait is not always unsteady, nor the tongue always tremulous; but if the coincidence of the physical symptoms is sometimes broken, their concurrent absence never occurs. Rarely more than one of the symptoms is absent, and enough remains to render the group pathognomonic.

This is all I shall at present say regarding the physical signs of general paralysis, reserving for a future occasion (page 27) a particular notice of each symptom.

Mental Symptoms of General Paralysis in its Second Stage.

The mental conditions that accompany these physical signs are various, but may be referred to one of three classes, namely—1st, elation, with large delusions; 2dly, depression, with melancholic delusions; 3dly, incomplete dementia, without delusion, and sometimes without incoherence.

The first class, that of elation with large delusions, is by far the most remarkable, as it is unlike any other phase of insanity. It has, from its prominence, so fixed the attention and filled the minds of some observers, that they have asserted that general paralysis is always, and exclusively, accompanied by it, an opinion from which the arrangement of the subject sufficiently shows how entirely I dissent.

Paralytic elation varies in every case, and includes every form of exaltation of the spirits, from mere quiet joyousness and self-complacency to the most boisterous mirth and noisiest demonstration of inward satisfaction of which human lungs and human gestures are capable. This elation is, in a large majority of cases, accompanied by excitement, which not infrequently rises into the most furious mania. The particular mode of exhibition varies with the individual, and may possibly be affected by his personal bias. The paralytic evinces his gladness by the same instinctive demonstrations as obtain among the sane. The lighthearted intuitively, without consulting their will, find themselves singing, or at least

making some sound more or less musical. So a common
evidence of paralytic elation is its subject, who probably
has never before shown any particular pleasure in music,
suddenly surprising his friends by his boisterous singing.
A hitherto decorous man, and not previously addicted to
psalmody, annoys the congregation by bawling out the
Psalm tunes ; or he astonishes his family by sending
home musical instruments, which he sets about learning
with great enthusiasm but little success.

He seems to see everything through a captivating
medium, which magnifies the importance of every trifle
he feverishly pursues. All looks to him rose-coloured.
He adopts with ardour every pseudo-science of which
our age is so prolific, and, if a medical man, is perhaps
in turn vegetarian, homœopath, and chronothermalist.

He is full of all manner of schemes, many of which,
though not quite mad, are only not so, because their
success is not physically impossible. He enters upon
these with an impetuous imprudence, which speedily
renders him the victim of the first unscrupulous person
he has to deal with. Impelled onward by his spirits,
and clad in the reason-proof panoply of self-sufficiency
he is at once too confident and too confiding.

A married man, who had hitherto observed the
decencies of life, openly keeps a mistress ; a heretofore
prudent and sagacious tradesman is on a sudden nearly
entrapped into a glaringly disreputable marriage. A
surgeon of small means and practice adds a horse to his
equipage, and dresses himself in gayer colours than had
hitherto been usual with him. A country practitioner,
a man of talent and of a studious turn, suddenly buys
and attentively reads penny song-books and the lightest
of ephemeral prints. An assistant-surgeon takes to

riding his employer's horses at such a furious rate, that
an accident compels him to leave his situation. A well-
educated, business-like grocer startles the town by the
sudden grandiloquence of his advertisements. Self-
satisfaction is visible in every look and every gesture, and
the gait alone, from its jaunty complacency, is frequently
sufficient to characterise the malady.

All these extravagant vagaries are not more extravagant than many which men at large, and considered sane,
are frequently guilty of; it is the gradual or sudden
change from sobriety of idea, demeanour, and conduct, to
frivolity, levity, and recklessless which stamps the disease
and marks its progress.

This mixture of elation and self-sufficiency increasing,
rapidly brings their subject to the confines of extravagant
delusion. The transition from the half-mad schemer to
the imaginary capitalist is natural; he now talks of the
wealth he fancies his projects have brought him.

A German physician who, after many vicissitudes,
had embarked his all in a commercial partnership in
London, into which he was cheated while in the first
stage, and who performed all the drudgery of the desk
and even of the warehouse, began to fancy he was
possessed of numerous offices, and of a large staff of
clerks and porters : a bachelor, he fancied he was
married, described the beauty of his wife, and talked of
his nineteen children. A poor widow from a workhouse
imagined she had married her surgeon, that she had
had several children by him, and insisted on remaining
in bed a fortnight after her supposed delivery. A coach-
man from Brighton informed his attendant he had been
the day before examined by twenty doctors. A lady,
who had been twelve months in an asylum, fancied she

had been there ninety years, and that she was "getting on for 200." An Indian soldier imagined he was 200 years old. A lady caressed her pillow for an infant, of which she thought she had been lately brought to bed. Our singing paralytic plans a voyage to Australia, whence he proposes sending £100,000 during the first month to his parents. Our galloping assistant-surgeon imagines a duke has sent for him to be his domestic medical attendant, and has in consequence settled a large pension on him. A crippled fan-piercer imagines Prince Albert is his brother, and asserts with glee he has " four millions of money." A bankrupt grocer talks of his large estate and noble descent. A poor fisherman fancies "all the ships at Spithead" belong to him. A gardener's wife announces herself as the rose of Waltham; and a frightfully attenuated servant asks you to admire her pretty hands and face.

But paralytic elation does not stop here; the whirl of the spirits increases, and self-complacency rises into self-translation and fancied supereminence. As the paralytic's estate and condition had been too lowly for him, now his very existence in his real name and station are intolerable. He denies, or rather he disbelieves, his identity. Our German physician becomes the brother of Sir John Franklin; a journeyman printer styles himself the Prophet Daniel; the Indian soldier has become Christ, and the bankrupt grocer calls himself God; a porter's wife calls herself a "little queen;" the lady "getting on for 200" has become a peer's daughter, and imagines her aunt is a marchioness; the "Rose of Waltham" is now a Queen of England, and boisterously asserts that God is the father of her children.

Arrived at this pitch, everything becomes invested with

immensity, grandeur, or beauty. Common pebbles are transformed into gems, and hoarded accordingly; the linen sheets become velvet, a white-washed wall silver, and a chamber utensil gold; "the little queen" makes queens of her sisters; the journeyman printer calls his medical attendant "that great and glorious man the Apostle Philip;" a ruined farmer imagines all his neighbours are a 1000 years old; an aged paralytic calls her sitting-room a palace, and her doctor Prince Albert; and our fan-piercer asserts that he has on his bed "160 quilts, 96 blankets, and 21 sheets." This condition of things does not remain stationary; the effervescence of the spirits either subsides, or markedly increases. The delusions gradually fade, or are speedily augmented. In the former case the patient sinks into a state of dementia more or less complete; in the latter the mental symptoms are aggravated till the maniacal fury becomes of the most intense character. Incessantly talking and restless, violent and destructive, tearing everything tearable to shreds, sleepless, dirty in his habits, and taking his food reluctantly, the paralytic rapidly becomes so attenuated, feeble and physically wretched, as to present as piteous a spectacle as human misery can offer. He lies on his bed feebly tearing his sheets, or on the padded floor of his room in a dream of happiness and splendour, which contrasts horribly with his hollow features and emaciated, squalid body. Happily death is at hand—exhaustion or paralytic coma soon closes the scene.

THE SECOND GROUP OF MENTAL SYMPTOMS, accompanying the second stage of general paralysis, comprises numerous cases in which the depression of the spirits is marked, and the delusions are of a decidedly melancholic type. This group is not so characteristic of the disease as that of elation. It may be mistaken for mere melancholia, while paralytic exaltation can with difficulty be confounded with any other form of madness. The manifestations of depression are probably as numerous, though scarcely so obtrusive, as those of exaltation. A bank-clerk imagined that his system was permeated by sugar of lead, and that poisons were entering his body by various inlets; a Scripture-reader, that he was accused of horrible crimes, and that he was kept in an asylum by a conspiracy of his friends; a fish-seller, that he had no tongue, mouth or limbs; and a poor woman, that her husband had been buried alive, and that nearly all her bones had been broken. A farm-labourer fancied he constantly heard voices repeating, " He is a thief, he is a scoundrel, he shall be hung;" an undertaker was extremely depressed and unhappy, because his meals, as he thought, were not paid for; a housemaid refused her food because she imagined she had committed inexpiable crimes, and was incessantly seeking a secluded spot wherein to destroy herself; a paralytic costermonger nearly killed himself by beating his head with a mallet, and subsequently his life was in danger from a self-inflicted cut-throat; a poor countrywoman never smiled, was silent, frequently in tears, and statuesque. A bricklayer imagined he was poisoned by foul gases in the street, and in consequence immured himself strictly in his house; a skipper attempted to throw himself into the Surrey Canal; and a Cambridgeshire labourer was very depressed, incessantly restless, and fancied he was the devil.

Slight depression, with great irritability of temper, moroseness, impulsive scurrility, and a remarkable turn for false accusation, are frequent mental combinations in this malady. An old lady, always morose and irritable, would sometimes bite, scratch, and swear fearfully. A Sussex woman was impulsively abusive, and had a long defamatory history to tell of all her fellow patients. A veterinary surgeon would, without provocation, write to his wife the most insulting letters, and on the most trivial occasions pour forth a torrent of abusive epithets, and put himself into fighting attitudes. An Essex labourer, who never smiled and was extremely morose, in a savage impulse seriously injured his attendant. An heraldic painter was intensely irritable, and without cause suddenly attacked his fellow patients with extreme violence.

The physical wear and tear attendant on this second group of mental symptoms of the paralysed, is infinitely less than the rapid prostration and exhaustion of the elated group. While in the latter the duration of the disease rarely exceeds two or three years, and is frequently fatal in a few months; in the former the depressed or morose paralytic drags on a very tolerable existence during many years.

When the melancholic delusions are of a very fearful character, the patient sometimes rapidly succumbs, but more frequently sinks into a state of more or less complete dementia.

It is difficult to conceive that an elated and a depressed mental condition can be contemporaneous in the same person; yet there are instances in which the delusions—the result, as I believe, of these diseased emotions—are certainly tinged by both, though the hue of the one or other predominates. Thus, a paralytic blacksmith, who was completely incoherent and usually cheerful, had an extraordinary mixed delusion, in which exaltation was, however, clearly in the ascendant; he fancied he went into the clouds every night, where he saw millions of beautiful female forms, many of which, however, had lost their arms, legs, breasts, and heads. A pilot's wife, who, imagining she was Queen of Denmark, talked incessantly of " his royal highness in scarlet" and of " her ministerialists," jumbled these lofty topics with the most virulent abuse, with spitefulness, and the oddest false accusations of injury to herself.

Though actual contemporaneity of exaltation and depression but rarely occurs, an alternation of these conditions is by no means uncommon, and the delusions, for the time being, are clearly referable to one only of these emotions. Sometimes the alternations follow no particular order, and the mental symptoms, though paroxysmal, are neither regular in their periods, nor equal in their intensity. A peculiar type of delusion is not *strictly* maintained, although the general tenor of the mental symptoms, and the prevailing colouring of the diseased ideas, are sufficiently evident. The usually elated paralytic may now and then, for a few days or hours, become the subject of melancholic fancies ; or, depressed, he may burst from his sadness into a fleeting gleam of joyous madness. A railway employé was usually depressed. He then fancied " all the world was on the verge of ruin; that not an acre of good land existed in the United Kingdom; and that the proprietors of railway and canal shares would all be ruined, the fares they charged being inadequate to recompense the companies for the original outlay of £1000 a foot." When very low, he asserted, with tears in his eyes, that the " Queen and all the lords had been massacred in Palace Yard." At these periods he refused food, or at most took it but sparingly. At rare intervals, however, he expressed himself as "very jolly." He then imagined himself the "most wonderful person living," and that, in consequence of having a galvanic machine in his thorax, he should live for ever. Convinced of this delusion, he was particularly anxious to engage himself as an exhibition to Mr. Albert Smith, and wished that a private entrance should be made for her Majesty, whom he expected among his earliest visitors. This casual abeyance of misery was evident through the nearly complete dementia in which he passed the last two months of life.

Sometimes the alternating melancholia and elated mania are as remarkable for precision of paroxysm and interval as some instances of recurrent mania. It is difficult to say which condition predominates. The alternations occur usually at short or long, rarely at medium, intervals. Thus, paralytic melancholia frequently lasts two or three days, and two or three months, more rarely two or three weeks. At the expiration of the low stage, a similar period of elated mania supervenes. Where the vicissitude is tertian or quartan, it may go on for months or years. When, however, the alternating paroxysm is an affair of three or four months, and especially if each phase be maniacal, the ordinary duration of the disease does not permit of their frequent recurrence. Between the paroxysms a period of uncertain length is frequently observed, during which actual or comparative tranquillity or sanity obtains.

Our German doctor, who imagined he was Sir John Franklin's brother and the father of nineteen children, completely recovered from these delusions. In sixteen weeks his elated spirits had become equable, and the only recognisable psychical symptom that remained was greatly impaired memory, which was principally evident in the comparative oblivion of his native tongue. During this improved state he was sent home to his friends. In sixty-two days from his discharge he returned to the asylum. He was now greatly depressed and very apprehensive, imagining that he was pursued by the police, that the upper part of his sister-in-law's house was on fire, and that the lower floor was deluged by a flood. He cowered in corners to escape pursuit, and never smiled. For a week he remained in this state, then had an attack of pure catalepsy, after which he became utterly demented, and in five weeks died of exhaustion. A poor woman from Brighton, admitted in February, 1851, was not then recognised as a paralytic. She remained stupid and depressed till January 3d, 1853, when she had a fit with complete hemiplegia sinistra; from this in a month she had quite recovered. From November 1853, to April, 1854 (the date of her death), she was every two or three days merry and incoherently talkative, or extremely depressed and taciturn. Though she had no marked delusions, the difference of these two states was very singular. During these six months she had several complete paralytic attacks; and when, after each seizure, she had recovered her consciousness, but not her utterance, she expressed her alternating feelings by tears or smiles. A tailor's wife, admitted January 3d, 1854, was very elated, and fancied she was married to three husbands. During the first two months of her residence, supposing she had had two children, she insisted on remaining in bed after each supposed birth. In November, 1854, she became morose, discontented, and imagining her food was drugged, thrust it away with violence; she abused her attendant, and accused her of poisoning it.

A ruined publican, when admitted in February, 1854, was morose, and had no large ideas. After a month or two he became cheerful and amiable, and fancied that, having lost eight millions of money, he had recovered it by advertising. Towards October, he again became morose, and remained so till he died, in November, 1854.

A Scotch sailor, when admitted in the autumn of 1852, imagined that his food was poisoned, and that his drink was depraved by "spirits." He was depressed and irritable. Sometimes he fancied that, in consequence of breathing twelve different gases, he was compelled to adopt as many modes of action. From June to September, 1853 (when he was removed), he was cheerful and well-conducted. During these three months his delusions were enormous; he was now constantly asserting that he had two millions and a half of money, and liberally offered £400,000 to his medical attendant to connive at his escape.

THE THIRD GROUP OF MENTAL SYMPTOMS attendant on this, the second stage of general paralysis, is incomplete dementia, usually without incoherence, and apparently unaccompanied by delusion. It is the absence of delusion which entitles this mental condition to be classed separately, and as such to merit a distinct notice; for dementia, more or less complete, is a symptom of all varieties and all stages of the disease. This incomplete dementia is characterised by a diminished capability of the purely intellectual powers. The perception of ideas appears to be blunted; an idea, which the paralytic would have formerly grasped at once, now eludes him, or takes him some time and trouble to master; or it may be that he seizes the idea, but, having perceived it, is indifferent to it. The memory fails. In marked cases this is easy enough to make out, but not always so easy when the patient is a stranger, and the failing not signal. To the friends of the patient it is much less difficult; they know the natural capacity of his retentive power, and can therefore calculate, with something approaching accuracy, the epoch and rate of its decay.

The faculty of the attention may be merely enfeebled, or nearly in abeyance. The patient's thoughts may widely wander, but still be capable of recall, or he may have completely lost the power of keeping ideas steadily before him.

With blunted perception, failing memory, and wandering attention, the process of comparing and combining ideas, of selecting those apposite to a subject, and of evoking a conclusion, must be (to say the least of it) difficult. The ratiocination of the paralytic is therefore imperfect, or rather, from the necessary preliminaries failing him, he is nearly incapable of exercising the act on any subject of even moderate importance. By this mental decay he is rendered incapable of retaining his social position, or of following his vocation. The abstraction and mistakes of the professional man or tradesman soon become too glaring not to convince his clientelle, of his unfitness to transact their business; and the artisan, though he may follow his calling longer, soon loses his skill and his customers.

The state of the spirits varies in this mental condition, but depending apparently on the naturally gay or sombre character of the patient, he is neither more elated or more melancholy than in health.

Having thus described the three distinct forms of mental alienation which accompany the second stage of general paralysis, I will mention some mental symptoms which are common to them all.

The most usual immediate cause of the paralytic's admission into an asylum is his extreme and sudden violence; and it commonly happens that his wife or some immediate relative is the intended victim or actually injured person. That this dangerous violence is frequently the consequence of delusion is certain; in rarer cases, however, no apposite delusion being discoverable, we are left to fall back on mere impulse for its explanation.

A married paralytic concealed under his pillow an open knife; another, who fancied his wife unfaithful, in an attempt to get at her, smashed doors and windows, and would have murdered her, had she not escaped from the house; a third, irritable, but free from delusion, frequently threatened his wife with the poker; a fourth, fancying his wife was conspiring against him, frequently threatened her life.

To that dangerous class of the community, wandering lunatics, the subjects of general paralysis largely contribute. Elated, full of schemes, and conscious of their sufficiency to grapple with every emergency; depressed and fleeing from some supposed danger or pursuit; or lost and wandering about purposeless; they form no mean proportion of the lunatics casual to all large towns or chargeable to counties.

Destructiveness is another very usual symptom or mental emanation of the paralysed. This propensity, as far as I can discover, is oftener dictated by impulse than by delusion. The habit of collecting rubbish, and of secreting it about the person, is frequently observed. Delusion appears to be sometimes the cause of this propensity, which is often very remarkable; thus, a poor surgeon would fill his pockets with stones, mistaking them for rubies; and, at once destructive and patriotic, broke twigs off the bushes and, sticking them in the ground at regular distances, imagined he was planting a forest of oaks for the navy.

But the most remarkable symptom, common to all forms of general paralysis, is a sudden accession of excitement, which speedily gains intensity, and often rises to the height of the most furious mania. This sudden excitement, in the majority of cases, commences in, and is confined to the night. If it persist through the day, an exacerbation will be unmistakeably observed towards evening. This usually occurs in the early hours of the night, generally before midnight.

At these periods, and in the worst cases, noise, restlessness, dirty, destructive habits, and maniacal raving, are all carried to an extreme pitch. I have seen no mania comparable with paralytic furor. Sheets, blankets, clothes, are all torn to shreds, the walls and bedsteads are plastered with excrement, and the poor patient wanders restlessly about his room, seeking some new object to destroy. Towards morning he becomes calm, sleeps, and in the day appears quite tranquil. These accessions do not occur nightly, or, if so, only for a few consecutive nights; nor are they all of so violent a character as those just described. In the depressed form they are sometimes welcomed by the patient and his attendants, for they simulate that mitigation of misery which is so usual towards evening among melancholics.

It is at night that the paralytic, when at large, usually attacks his immediate attendants. He is no doubt impelled to violence by his nocturnal maniacal paroxysm.

Mental Symptoms of the Third Stage of General Paralysis.

The mental condition of the paralysed during the third and last stage of their malady is indeed deplorable. It is that of complete dementia. This third stage, however, he does not always attain.

In the second stage, as I have before shown, he frequently succumbs under the intense excitement which usually accompanies the elated form of the disease. A paralytic seizure may be fatal to him long before complete dementia has set in; and accidents, to which, from his mental decay and unsteady gait, he is very liable, or any of the common acute diseases, to which his feeble constitutional powers can offer but slight resistance, may suddenly terminate his existence at any period of the disease.

If he arrive at this last condition, he is a complete mental wreck. Physically feeble, he totters about without an object; from mere lostness he is dirty in his habits; laying his hands mechanically on everything within his reach, he instinctively pockets it, without knowing its use, value or name; languidly destructive, his memory annihilated, his speech unintelligible and only heard at long intervals, he appears to have attained the lowest depth of intellectual degradation.

During genial weather the demented paralytic may pass a tolerable existence, but nipped by the first cold day, or stricken by any disease, however slight, all his symptoms increase. A trifling attack of bronchitis or diarrhœa will carry him off. If bedridden, a sudden change of posture, from the horizontal to the erect, brings him to the verge of existence—a palsy-shake or a bed-sore pushes him over it.

Strange though it may appear, it is often in this, the third stage, that the disease is for the first time recognised. From parish workhouses, and even from respectable wealthy homes, comes many a poor demented paralytic, with his head shaved, his nape blistered, with leech-bites on his temples and cupping marks on his shoulders; his wrists and ankles abraded or ulcerated from restraint, his abdomen discoloured from having been bound to his bed by a sheet; emaciated to the last degree, his trochanters nearly starting through the tense livid skin, with bed-sores over the sacrum and on the nates, and with the inguinal clefts excoriated by ammoniacal urine. He has been neglected by his domestic attendants, who have probably thought such an existence was not worth continuing; or he has been hurried into dementia and extremity by the fervour of his doctor, who has evidently imagined he had to deal with an acute and curable cerebral disease.

By a rigid hygiene, by scrupulous cleanliness, by a generous diet, he is sometimes partially redeemed from this pitiable plight, and may, in some rare instances, pass years of a tolerable physical existence, in a condition but little removed from complete dementia.

CHAPTER II.

A DETAILED ACCOUNT OF THE BODILY CONDITION AND PHYSICAL SYMPTOMS OF GENERAL PARALYSIS.

1. THE GENERAL CONDITION OF THE BODY is bad or good, as the excitement is intense or as a comparative tranquillity is maintained. The wear and tear of the exalted form of the malady is, as before mentioned, always greater than that of the depressed form; but it is not until great excitement supervenes upon either of these conditions that the bodily condition markedly declines. Then the patient rapidly emaciates. This loss of substance is the more remarkable, as it usually happens that, up to the date of the excitement, the patient has been gaining weight—flesh it would be inexact to say, for the increase appears to be owing to a diffused unhealthy fat, which rounds off all the angles of the body, and gives to the incipient paralytic a flabby sleekness, which his friends frequently mistake for the robust muscularity of health. On this imperfectly formed adeps the excited paralytic may be said sometimes wholly to subsist; for, from mental preoccupation, or from some extravagant exalted, or melancholic delusion, he frequently refuses food, or takes it with extreme reluctance and in small quantity.

The excitement and the emaciation advancing simultaneously, all the fat is absorbed, and the patient, if the excitement continue, soon realises the popular figure of a living skeleton. Should the excitement pass away spontaneously, or be subdued by treatment, the paralytic, if he be not too far gone, gradually regains his flabby condition. In that state he may remain for years, until another attack of excitement happens, or till, dementia advancing, he again gradually emaciates— a condition which, his organic nervous power completely failing, is speedily followed by death.

In the incompletely demented form of the malady, the sleek appearance of the patient is sometimes very remarkable, and it is only after a paralytic seizure or shake that emaciation ensues. From this seizure, or from many such, he frequently rapidly recovers, and only succumbs to nervous exhaustion coincident with complete dementia, or to a seizure of unusual severity.

2. The FACIAL EXPRESSION of the paralytic is peculiar. There is a stolid vacancy and a want of play of feature which, though not obtrusive symptoms, are, when attention has been called to them, very remarkable and easy of recognition. Though the patient is frequently agitated by the most stormy passions; though his delusions, whether of exaltation or depression, are peculiarly calculated to leave their impress on the face; yet it remains comparatively unmoved during moments or hours, while fury or maniacal joy, moroseness or depression, are only too evident from the actions, the gestures, or the language of the patient. The mouth, which contributes so much to the variety and colouring of expression, remains nearly fixed, and the whole mus-

cular machinery of facial expression is quiescent, and apparently incapable of being again set in motion by the ideas. The paralytic's lower jaw may descend in the act of laughing, but the reverse of Sardinian laughter is the result ; he laughs with his heart, but hardly with his face. The low adeps which is deposited in all other parts of the body is not absent from the face, and contributes to the vacant repose of the paralytic's features. From these two causes the face, in the second stage of the disease, is frequently described in the case-books as fat, pendulous, and expressionless.

In this facial apathy the eye does not participate. That organ still indicates the condition of the ideas, and its glances, irritable or savage, drooping or exalted, maintain, even in general paralysis, its reputation as the herald of the mind.

3. THE COMPLEXION varies greatly, according to the age of the patient, and the stage of the disease.

At the commencement of the second stage, and during the middle period of life (from thirty to fifty), the patient, coincident with his flabby sleekness, has frequently a brilliant scarlet colour, extending nearly all over the cheeks, the rest of the face retaining its usual tint. Of the victims of general paralysis the great majority are observed to be persons of light complexions, thin skins, and blue or gray eyes. Whether this circumstance arises from the greater number of such persons in Britain, or from any predisposition of the fair-complexioned, I do not at present feel myself competent to determine, though I strongly incline to the latter idea. The paralytic may give to the world the idea of a healthy person with a brilliant, florid complexion, but to the medical eye it is of too deep a colour. It is the re-sult of languid circulation; the least touch of the finger drives the colour from the point of contact, and it is some time—often many seconds—before the feeble arterial power, reinjecting the capillaries, restores its scarlet hue.

Among paralytics who have passed the middle age (fifty), the skin of the face sometimes presents a very singular appearance. It seems as if partially dried up; the brow and cheeks are deeply indented with hard, fixed lines, and the complexion is brownish and waxen. On looking at these faces, one is reminded of tinted creased parchment. If the patient be in tolerable health and spirits, the injected capillaries, shining through the waxen skin, give his face all the advantages of a brilliantly clear complexion, and the aspect of perfect health. If, on the contrary, he be depressed, feeble, or emaciated, the sallow corrugated skin gives him the look of haggard, squalid decrepitude. This parchmenty complexion, which is frequently also observed among recurrent maniacs, I have found invariably coincident with rigidity of the arteries, and usually with contracted and very sluggish pupils. Arterial rigidity may be very marked, and the skin of the face natural; but it has never happened to me to observe this parchment-like skin without the radial or brachial being distinctly rigid, and frequently tortuous. The vessel rolls under the finger like a piece of whipcord.

The face, towards the close of the malady, participates in the complete dementia and general physical wretchedness which accompany the last stage. It is yellow, wan, and expressionless.

4. PTOSIS is sometimes observed among the paralysed, but it is neither a common nor a marked sign.

5. THE CONDITION OF THE IRIS is perhaps the most remarkable, as it certainly is the most interesting, symptom of the disease—an interest, which the imperfect notice it has received from those otherwise conversant with the malady, has not diminished.

It may be broadly stated, that in all cases of general paralysis, at some epoch of the disease, the mobility of the irides is lessened, or their symmetry disturbed. In the great majority of instances, the diminished mobility, or damaged symmetry, is permanent, though it is rarely *equally* evident at all times. In some few cases, the symmetry and normal contractility are *commonly* maintained, but at uncertain periods either one or other of these markedly deviates from its usual condition. This may be considered a bold statement; it is at least one which can only be made or refuted by an attentive watcher.

At the risk of being deemed prolix, I will describe the various deviations from the normal pupillary condition which obtain in general paralysis. And first, of the pupillary forms arising from symmetrical contraction.

The most remarkable of these is that condition of the iris which has been aptly termed "the pin-point pupil." It is principally remarked during the first stage of the malady. The iris is firmly contracted to the size of a pin's point, and its mobility is destroyed, vision being unimpaired. This pin-point condition is rare. I have little doubt, however, that it will be ascertained to be one of the *earliest* symptoms of the first stage of general paralysis. The next form is that in which the iris is markedly contracted and motionless, though the contraction is less than in the pin-point condition. This symmetrical and permanent contraction is not uncommon. The cases in which the pupillary symmetry is not strictly maintained, nor the power of motion quite destroyed, are, however, far more frequently met with. In these examples the pupil is rarely round, but rather irregularly angular. The pupillary areæ may be equal, though the inner margin of the iris be slightly and dissimilarly irregular in both eyes. Sometimes the pupil is permanently midway between contraction and dilatation, very sluggish in its movements, trapezoidal or triangular, and not uniform in the two eyes. The inequality in these instances, though real, is trifling, and though it merit, does not compel, attention.

The second group of pupillary forms comprises those cases in which the want of symmetry is marked, concomitant contraction of the iris not being a leading feature. Thus, both pupils may be of moderate size, their margins round and regular, one, however, being clearly the larger. In many instances this disparity is most conspicuous. In some cases the affected pupil is obliquely flattened, so that the margin, though regular, is no longer round, but obliquely oval, elliptical, or gibbous. The axis of the pupil is by this flattening completely changed; instead of being directly backwards towards the bottom of the orbit, its direction is obliquely upwards and outwards, or more rarely upwards and inwards. For these altered pupillary axes, converging and diverging, appear appropriate terms. Now and then the pupil is flattened above and below, or laterally; whence result oval shapes with a horizontal or vertical axis. Occasionally the disparity is rendered remarkable by one pupil being strongly contracted and motionless, the other retaining its normal size and mobility. Where, however, one pupil is dilated and sluggish, the other being permanently contracted, the most remarkable deviation from pupillary symmetry obtains. A not unusual condition of the iridal margin is very peculiar. It suddenly juts out like a promontory into the expanse of the aqueous humour. There are sometimes several of these salient projections, sometimes only one. They might be easily mistaken for old iritic adhesions; that they are not so, is sufficiently proved by their sudden appearance, their sudden absence, and then as sudden return.

In some instances, when the difference of the pupillary areæ is not great, a regular margin being at the same time maintained in both eyes, it is not easy to discover which is the affected, or the more affected organ. If there were a normal mean pupillary area, it would be easy enough, by comparing the two pupils with the standard, to determine which was the more implicated. This, however, is so far from being the case, that the contractility of the iris under a given luminosity can scarcely be said to be the same in any two individuals; and it frequently varies in the same person according to his state of health, or even of spirits.

How then is the affected iris to be distinguished? By its diminished contractile power. That iris is the more affected whose motions are the more sluggish. If a general paralytic with equal pupils be taken into a darkened room, it will be seen that one pupil expands more freely in the dusk than the other. As long as the patient remains in the twilight, the disturbed symmetry is apparent. The less expanded is, of course, the more implicated pupil. Pupils that are equal in the patient's ordinary sitting-room, become unsymmetrical in the padded room, which is always somewhat darker.

This mode of determining the respective contractility of the irides is preferable, among paralytic lunatics at least, to the commonly adopted plan of using a lighted candle. The latter method, indeed, which is rarely advisable, is usually impossible : as, even if the patient be calm at the commencement of the examination, he speedily becomes excited during its progress.

Whenever marginal irregularity, or a changed axis exists, that I take to be the more implicated organ. Marked contraction, or marked dilatation of one iris sufficiently well tells its own tale, and of two irregular irides, the more irregular is doubtless the more damaged

I have been thus minute in describing the peculiarities of the iris in general paralysis, and thus circumstantial in pointing out the means of distinguishing the more affected pupil, as I believe, that with the state of the iris, the condition of the spirits, and consequently the tone of the delusions, are found to vary. From observations which have now extended over six years, during the earlier part of which I was gradually led to this inference, and during the latter part of which I have endeavoured to divest myself of preconception and the subject of every source of fallacy, I have become daily more convinced, from what I have daily witnessed, that depression of spirits and melancholic delusions are associated, among general paralytics, with affected right pupil; and that elation and grand or pleasurable fancies are associated with affected left pupil. By affection of the pupil, I do not mean any one peculiar condition of the iris; its inner circle may be contracted to a point, or its outer circle contracting peripherally, may, by extreme dilatation, be reduced to a narrow rim. The pupil may be markedly irregular, sluggish, or its axis may be evidently changed. That each of these conditions may in time be found to have a significance of its own, I think very probable. In the mean time, however, unable to distinguish these nice shades of diagnosis, I merely judge of the more implicated pupil by its more conspicuous contraction, dilatation, irregularity, or sluggishness. Where the pupils are slightly and equally affected, I have observed no delusion at all, and with equal and signal pupillary implication, alternating or mixed delusions. When both pupils have been evidently affected, but one rather the more so, mixed or alternating delusions have been usually remarked with a predominance of delusion, however, corresponding with the more implicated pupil. When the right pupil has been the more affected, the *general* tone of the delusions has been melancholic ; and with a more implicated left pupil, their *usual* complexion has been elated, and their colouring gorgeous. With these prefatory remarks, I enter on an analysis of *all* the cases of general paralysis, regarding the pupillary condition of which I have notes.

A tabular view of 100 unselected cases, showing the coincidence of affected right pupil and melancholic delusion, of affected left pupil and maniacal elation, and of slight and equal pupillary affection and freedom from delusion.

				OPINION		
				Against	Neutral regarding	In favour of
Of 29	Depressed male paralytics	26	Had affected right pupil			26
	,,	1	Had affected left pupil	1		
	,,	2	Had both pupils apparently equally affected		2	
Of 14	Depressed female paralytics	13	Had affected right pupil			13
	,,	1	Had both pupils equally affected		1	
Of 17	Elated male paralytics	11	Had affected left pupil			11
	,,	1	Had affected right pupil	1		
	,,	5	Had equal or equally affected pupils		5	
Of 4	Elated female paralytics	4	Had affected left pupil			4
Of 14	Male paralytics, with varying or mixed delusions in	6	The dilatation of the pupils varied with the delusions. When elated, or the subject of exalted delusions, the left pupil was the larger, or the pupils were equal. When dejected or oppressed by melancholic fancies, the right was the larger			6

		Description			
6		Male paralytics, with varying or mixed delusions in — (Including two cases of mixed delusions) both pupils were equally affected. If these cases had been more closely watched, the condition of the pupils would probably have been found varying with the delusions	6	—	2
2	Of 8	,, in — Both pupils were affected, but one the more markedly. The predominance of delusion corresponded with the more implicated pupil	2	—	—
6		Female paralytics, with alternating delusions in — The condition of the pupils varied with that of the spirits, and with the delusions	6	—	—
2		,, in — Both pupils were equally affected. If these cases had been more attentively watched, the condition of the pupil would probably have been found varying with that of the spirits, and with the delusions	2	—	—
7	Of 9	Male paralytics who had no delusion, and whose spirits were unaffected, but who were all demented or semi-demented in — The pupils were equally, but not signally, affected	7	—	—
2		,, in — Though both pupils were affected, one was slightly the more so	—	2	—
3	Of 5	Female paralytics, who had no delusion or affection of the spirits in — The pupils were equally, but not signally, affected	3	—	—
2		,, in — Though both were affected, one was slightly the more so	—	2	—
100			**86**	**12**	**2**

A rule, that in a hundred *unselected* cases has but two exceptions, hardly requires corroboration.

It is, however, directly confirmed by the *variations* of the unsymmetrical pupils. As I have before mentioned, the size of the affected iris is rarely uniform at every epoch of the disease. This variation I have found concurrent with changes of the spirits and ideas. A depressed paralytic with a slightly dilated right pupil becomes more melancholic, and his delusions of a lower or more horrible type. The slightly dilated right pupil enlarges. The increased depression passes away, and the paralytic returns to his mere usual melancholy. The pupil recedes to its former slight dilatation.

He becomes less depressed, or even a gleam of natural hilarity surprises him; the inequality, slight at first, entirely disappears, to return, however, on his speedy relapse into misery.

An exalted paralytic becomes more exalted: his left pupil, already the larger, enlarges. His spirits and delusions recede; the iris contracts to its former dimensions.

Convincing and instructive proofs of the truth of my opinion are to be found among those cases in which the pupils are usually symmetrical. These paralytics occasionally, without known cause, have sudden accessions of their melancholy or exaltation. In the former case the right, in the latter the left pupil dilates, and in proportion to the intensity of the diseased emotions: symmetry returns with the usual mental condition. The rare instances of the pupils alternating at short intervals (two or three days) in a most remarkable manner confirm the opinion. The spirits and ideas alternate in company with the irides.

Strong collateral evidence may be obtained from cases of insanity, which are not suspected of paralytic complication. This support is especially to be found among the class of recurrent or paroxysmal lunatics. Of these, there are many in whom the insane symptoms are of a very mild type. Rarely approaching glaring delusions, they consist in alternating depression and excited exaltation. This is insanity of the spirits rather than of the intellect; though any one, who has watched his own sensations, needs no telling how the intelligence is obscured by dejection, and brightened by cheerfulness. Among this class I have often observed that, during the many months which the depression frequently lasts, the right pupil has been the larger, and that, on its departure and the advent of the elated stage, the symmetry has been restored, not to be disturbed till the next period of depression. In cases of periodical elation, the left pupil is frequently found slightly but distinctly the larger.

This coincidence of dilated left pupil and exuberance of spirits is not so usual as that of dilated right pupil and depression; and it rarely happens that, in the same person, both periodical conditions are attended by corresponding pupillary changes. In recurrent mania, especially when accompanied, as it frequently is, by rigid arteries, the pupils are often contracted and very feebly sensitive. In the maniacal melancholia of old persons (especially women), whose arteries are nearly always rigid, the right pupil is frequently observed to be the larger and the more sluggish, or contracted and insensible.

As illustrative of the subject, I may briefly mention a few cases out of a large number that have come under my notice. I have notes of seventy cases of insane

persons, not paralytics or epileptics, in whom both pupils
are either contracted. irregular, and sluggish, or in
whom iridal disparity, to a greater or less extent. occasionally exists.

A man servant, æt. 25, when admitted was depressed,
taciturn, and stationary in his habits. The *right* pupil
was the *larger, and vertically oval*. His depression
is at uncertain intervals replaced by restless excitement and by noisy incoherent elation. The pupils are
now equal. The symmetry, however, only lasts during
the exalted fit. With the depression returns the inequality.

A tailor, æt. 19, when admitted was depressed,
taciturn, and solitary. Soon all his symptoms increased.
He became silent, statuesque and nearly cataleptic,
refused his food, and was the picture of the completest
apathy. During this time the *right* pupil was distinctly
the *larger*. The low symptoms very gradually passed
away, and were replaced by a condition of excited,
restless, but coherent joyousness. He was now industrious at his trade, sang, and amused himself rationally.
The pupils became nearly equal. The right, however,
was still usually rather the larger, though on many
occasions no difference was perceptible. Again he
relapsed into his depression, though to a much less
degree than heretofore. The right pupil was now
markedly the larger.

A labourer, æt. 30, is the subject of paroxysms of
excitement, during which he is utterly incoherent, and has
the grandest delusions. He calls himself the " Patriarch

Isaac," a king, God, and imagines he can command the firmament. At these periods his *left* pupil is markedly the *larger*. Gradually he becomes coherent, and his delusions vanish. The pupils have become equal, and remain so till the next paroxysm.

A farm labourer, æt. 37, usually morose, solitary, reserved and taciturn, but with no evident delusion, becomes at times elated, restless, and full of grand delusions. He now fancies he " owns the world," that he has large sums in the Bank of England, of which he liberally offers £1000 to his attendant to " get him out," and talks familiarly of " Prince Albert." His *left* pupil is now markedly the *larger*. His lofty fit passes away, and with it the disparity.

A lady, æt. 35, is admitted, restless, incoherent, and apprehensive, fancying that her son is dead, that those about her are plotting to injure her, and that some undefinable calamity is imminent. The *right* pupil is markedly the *larger and vertically oval*. She recovers her cheerfulness, but her apprehensions still hang about her. The right pupil, though still the larger, is much less so.

She is discharged by the order of her friends. In a fortnight she returns in the same apprehensive, depressed condition. The right pupil is now much the larger. In a day or two she gets better : when suddenly she is found in an intently listening attitude : she hears the sounds, " Your son is dead," and fancies a man, concealed in a ventilator, says, " I wish you to die," and "to have your dinner." While relating all this, she abruptly breaks off with a shriek, that " the devil is up her arm." The right pupil continues markedly the larger. She gradually regained her spirits and lost her delusions. Her suspicious fearfulness, however, though she did her best to subdue or to conceal it, was sometimes sufficiently evident. In this condition she was removed, the right pupil still remaining somewhat the larger.

A poor widow, æt. 54, borne down by labour and privation, is admitted in February, 1854, in a state of maniacal melancholia. She is extremely depressed and full of the most horrible fancies, imagines she is immediately to be killed, and is incessantly restless and trying to escape from her fancied pursuers.

The *right* pupil is the *larger*, and has a *diverging axis*.

Her delusions become more horrible, and her misery so great, that to lighten it she tears the sheets to shreds with her teeth, and gnaws the wood of her night-chair. She sometimes imagines that the whole " National debt" has been " incurred on her account." The dilatation of the right pupil increases, and remains so till November, 1854, when, worn out by her misery, she expires of exhaustion. In this case the radial and brachial were markedly rigid and tortuous.

A poor countrywoman, æt. 67, admitted July, 1853, was very depressed, and apprehensive she would never recover. The pupils were equal, and the arteries rigid. At first industrious, she at length became so depressed, as to be compelled to relinquish her occupation of laundress. The *right* pupil was now clearly the *larger*. Her spirits returned, but fearfulness, though much mitigated, remained. The inequality was now less marked : but an increase of depression reproduced it in its former conspicuousness.

A countrywoman, æt. 64, admitted July, 1854, was extremely dejected, and fancied she was doomed to perdition, though she was unable to say how she was worse than her neighbours. The condition of the pupils on admission was not recorded. The arteries were rigid. She regained her spirits, which indeed soon became too high. This elation without incoherence or delusion was succeeded by depression, during which the *right* pupil was clearly the *larger*. On the return of the elated stage the disparity disappeared.

A widow, æt. 67, a recurrent lunatic since 1842, whose alternating paroxysms of elation and depression are very remarkable, has the *left pupil enlarged* during the high stage. The arteries are rigid in this case.

A married woman, æt. 36, and in good health, was admitted in May, 1852, and has been a recurrent maniac ever since. During the lucid intervals she is coherent and well-conducted, though depressed. The *right pupil* is now markedly the *larger*. During the paroxysm she is highly excited, incoherent, restless, nymphomanic, and in the highest spirits. The pupils are now often equal, or nearly so, by the contraction of the dilated right pupil to the normal size of the left.

6. THE LIPS AND MOUTH OF GENERAL PARALYTICS are always more or less affected.

The mouth is usually closed and slightly compressed. The upper lip is straight, and its central depression and the curves thence arising, are frequently obliterated— always diminished. The curves of the lower lip are similarly changed. Both lips look as if pulled out or stretched, as in the act of laughing, the angles of the mouth, however, not being directed upwards, but extended horizontally.

This extension of the lips makes the mouth broader than heretofore; and with its horizontal and nearly immoveable angles, mainly produces the fixed, stolid expression of the paralytic's face. The change in the condition of the mouth is probably among the earliest symptoms of the disease. When the malady is far advanced, the lips, particularly the upper lip, are tremulous, as if with passion, and twitch slightly. This symptom is always more evident during the paroxysms of intense excitement, which are so characteristic of the disease. The symmetry of the mouth is usually maintained; though immediately after the evanescent hemiplegic seizures, which are of so frequent occurrence among general paralytics, the mouth is sometimes drawn to the side not paralysed, by the destruction of the equilibrium of the labial muscles.

7. GRINDING OF THE TEETH is of frequent occurrence among the paralysed, and is, as far as I know, to be observed among no other class of the insane.

Though rare in the early stage, and during the excitement, it is common during the later and demented, or semi-demented period. The poor half-lost madman sits for hours unconsciously grinding his teeth. If he be told of it, he usually denies the fact, and if at length convinced of the habit, owns his helplessness to prevent it. The front teeth in these persons are frequently worn down by incessant attrition.

The incipiently demented sometimes become suddenly stupid, stationary, and in a condition approaching semi-coma. Their gait is feeble and tottering, their lips tremulous, and their utterance very imperfect. They are on the verge of a seizure, which, however, is frequently avertible by a very simple treatment, which I shall presently mention. With these symptoms the most marked teeth-grinding is frequently associated, and with them disappears.

During the last period of the malady, the grinding of the teeth is to the attendants a most distressing symptom. To stand in an asylum infirmary, in which are three or four bedridden paralytics, to regard their sleeping, motionless forms, the silence of the night unbroken but by their loud monotonous teeth-grinding, is to witness a sight not easily forgotten, and to hear sounds indescribably awful and discordant.

8. The condition of the tongue varies greatly with the epoch of the disease. Of its condition in the first stage I have no experience. At the commencement of the second stage it is nearly constantly rather tremulous, largeish, somewhat paler and more flabby than usual, and frequently covered with a slight white fur. As the disease advances the tongue becomes more tremulous; it enlarges laterally, and seems to fill the mouth, the angles of which it stretches when protruded. The flabbiness increases, and the slight fur disappearing, the surface is left morbidly clean, and of a livid, pinkish colour. This state of the organ is very characteristic of the disease. The surface looks perfectly smooth, as if the epithelium and papillæ had been removed. Occasionally a few transverse, irregular rugæ are to be seen.

In the last stage the *tremor* is most marked; from this cause the tongue can frequently be not protruded, though the patient tries his hardest to do so, from inability to direct the tip to the aperture of the lips.

The tongue is, in a few cases, protruded slightly out of the mesian line, the tip being directed towards the paralysed side, in consequence of the balanced action of the opposite posterior lingual and pharangeal muscles being destroyed.

9. THE MOBILITY OF THE PHARANGEAL MUSCLES is towards the close of the malady most evidently diminished, and the reflex act of deglutition can be with difficulty performed. The sensibility of the pharangeal nerves is doubtless lessened, but this diminution does not approach anæsthesia so nearly as the lessened mobility approaches paralysis.

In former times, when asylums were less carefully superintended than at present, when knives and forks were denied the insane, when, their food not being cut for them, they were allowed to tear off a large morsel with their hands, and thrust it voraciously into their mouths, the poor paralytic was sometimes killed by the impaction of a morsel in the pharynx, and often brought to the verge of suffocation, from which he was only saved by his attendant promptly thrusting his hand into the pharynx and extricating the compressing body. Probangs, and long curved forceps to extract the lump, were everywhere at hand. They are now happily rarely required. In this condition, unable to keep up a continuous descending current in the œsophagus, the advanced paralytic takes liquid food, not at a draught, but in small, distinct, spasmodic gulps.

10. A DEFECTIVE UTTERANCE is one of the earliest

and most consistent signs of the second stage of general paralysis—a circumstance for which the tongue-trembling naturally prepares us. Though very usual, this symptom is not invariable. Indeed, in the worst case, perhaps, I ever saw, the articulation, though very peculiar from its measured, mincing affectation, was certainly very distinct and perfect.

The defect, in the commencement of the second stage, sometimes amounts to a mere trifling hesitation in the speech, and which, unaccompanied by other symptoms, would easily escape, and indeed, would scarcely deserve notice. The voice seems to linger over the syllables of a word. The disease advancing, the hesitation becomes a complete halt. During a minute, though perfectly appreciable space of time, the paralytic stops between the words of the current sentence, or the syllables of a word. The correct enunciation of long words is difficult, and only to be attained after repeated trials. Vowels are easily pronounced, but a word of many syllables, some of which commence with different, but *not very dissimilar* consonants, or with double consonants, foils the paralytic. He jumbles the somewhat similar and omits one of the double consonants. Thus, if asked to say "trigonometrical," he will say "trigo*m*ometrical," or "trigonome*t*ical," or any other collection of syllabic sounds than the correct. As the physical defect and mental decline advance simultaneously, the failing memory and diminished power of recall for ideas and words play their parts in the confused and halting utterance. The patient speaks slowly and with many breaks, because the simplest arrangement of ideas is a labour to him, or because, though the ideas are clear to him, he cannot recollect their verbal exponents. Thus, if he have two fruits placed before him, strawberries and cherries, he will sometimes call cherries strawberries, and *vice versá;* that this is from forgetfulness of the proper terms, and not from delusion, is abundantly clear from the fact, that as soon as the mistake is pointed out, the patient instantly recognises the error of appellation. The same remark applies to the proper names of persons.

During the last stage, when the tongue-trembling and pharangeal paralysis have become very marked, the articulation is so much impaired, that speech is with difficulty intelligible. Sometimes the paralytic, from absence of ideas, or physical inability to express them, is quite silent. During, however, the nocturnal exacerbations of excitement, the tongue, or at least the larynx, under this temporary fillip, appears to be loosened; for the paralytic will, for hours together, pour forth a torrent of half-shaped words or hideous noises, which render his society peculiarly unpleasant.

11. The Gait of general paralysis varies with the stage of the disease. At the commencement of the second stage, it is sometimes natural, but more frequently straddling. Though the paralytic be unaware of the feebleness of his lower extremities, instinct teaches him to compensate for it by increasing the width of the base of the triangle, the sides of which are formed by the legs. As the disease advances, the gait becomes devious, the paralytic is unable to walk straight, but has a shambling roll, which is very characteristic. When the delusions are magnificent and flattering to his vanity, he walks with a lofty, self-complacent air, which is rarely seen in any other form of insanity, and which contrasts forcibly with the evident

feebleness of the lower limbs. When the third stage is attained, that of dementia and of great physical feebleness, the straddle increases in width, and the roll becomes a totter. Occasionally in the low mental form of the malady, the patient will not or cannot walk, because he is impressed with the idea that he has no legs. It is sometimes possible to make out which is the more paralyzed leg, by a slight drag of the foot. Much more frequently, however, the equal feebleness of the legs demonstrates the impartiality or general character of the semi-paralysis.

12. THE PULSE of general paralysis is usually extremely feeble, and frequently, when the patient is tranquil, it can be with difficulty counted, or even felt. The cold livid hands and feet clearly enough indicate the langour of the circulation.

During the maniacal accessions, the pulse is not unfrequently thrilling, easily felt, but put out by the least pressure of the finger. It somewhat resembles the hæmorrhagic pulse, and gives one the idea of blood rushing swiftly through imperfectly-filled tubes.

When the arteries are rigid (as they are in at least 50 per cent. of general paralytics), the pulse is full and hardish. This deceptive *sensation* of power is evidently attributable to the *morbid density* of the arterial coats; in consequence of which the tube becomes a better conductor of vibrations, and so conveys the least pulsatile undulation with increased distinctness to the finger. The rigid radial and brachial roll under the finger like pieces of whipcord, and are often tortuous, a peculiarity which is likewise very observable in the anterior temporal arteries.

When rigidity has gone on to ossification, the pulse is annihilated, and the tube feels like a piece of rough wood or rope. This condition is very rare.

13. THE FITS which attend the majority of instances of general paralysis are remarkable and peculiar features —remarkable in common with all cognate seizures; peculiar, because, though often mistaken for apoplectic or epileptic fits, they are sufficiently distinct from either. These seizures are of three kinds—

1st. Those in which the coma is profound, the paralysis and anæsthesia complete and universal, and the abolition of reflex movements total.

2dly. Those in which hemiplegia is the most striking symptom, and in which anæsthesia and the destruction of the reflex movements are rarely complete. The coma is seldom profound, and the utterance, though at first in abeyance, soon regains an imperfect ascendancy.

3dly. Those in which, though the patient never becomes insensible, he is suddenly found stupid and bewildered, his memory destroyed, his utterance more halting, the gait more tottery and devious, the lips and tongue more tremulous than before.

Each of these seizures, though possible at any stage of the malady, has *usually* a distinct epoch and significance.

The first class of seizure, in which coma, paralysis, and anæsthesia are complete, is rarely observed, except as a concluding phenomenon of the disease. Worn out by his intense excitement, the poor insane paralytic is suddenly found perfectly comatose—a condition from which he rarely rallies. Immobility is unbroken, except by an occasional imperfect convulsion, by grinding of the teeth, or by a feeble rolling of the eyeball. Active treatment only hastens the approach of death : let alone, the patient frequently lasts four or five days.

The second class of seizure is by far the most frequent and remarkable. A *recognised* paralytic is suddenly found completely hemiplegic. I say " is found," for rarely is any one present, or, if present, cognisant of the exact time of the seizure. The fit, which usually happens in the night, is unattended by shriek or scream, and is frequently free from convulsion. It is accompanied by semi-coma and suspended utterance, and often announces itself to the attendants or to the hemiplegic's fellow-patients by loud teeth-grinding, or by the seized person falling out of bed. Then the neighbours find he has fallen because an arm and a leg are powerless. Frequently the paralytic, who may have been retained in bed by the well-tucked-in clothes, is only discovered to be hemiplegic when the attendant comes to get him up in the morning. It is at one of these periods that he comes under medical inspection.

He is now semi-comatose, his utterance is in abeyance, he is quite hemiplegic, but with sensation only slightly impaired. If the arm or leg be pinched, vigorous movements of the affected limbs ensue. Though sometimes apparently insensible to all going on around him, there is frequently a hopeful glimmer of intelligence in the eye. The mouth is rarely distorted, and the movements of the eyeball are more perfect than might be expected. The pupils are more unsymmetrical than usual.

The course of the narrative and the striking results of

a very simple treatment, make me here anticipate some of the little I have to say concerning the therapeutics of the disease. An attendant administers an injection of eight table-spoonfuls of common salt dissolved in a pint of warm water. In nine cases out of ten, in at most an hour, a copious stool is the result, composed of small, hard, quite distinct, rounded lumps. After an evacuation of this kind I have known a person quite hemiplegic at 2 p.m., recover a free mobility of the arm and leg by midnight. Usually, however, several similar enemata, and their resulting stools, are required before an approach to the ordinary movements of the limbs is obtained. Occasionally castor oil and a pill of two grains of calomel and three grains of Ext. Col. comp. are employed, the sooner to clear out the intestinal tube, or at least the large intestines.

The object of these simple remedies is not, by serous evacuations, to derive from the head, but simply to expel the hardened fæces, of which the colon is full, and which I regard as the eccentric cause of the seizure. The cause removed, nature, aided by a moderately generous diet, will soon restore the affected limbs to their former condition.

Any remedy producing copious serous motions is worse than useless; and, if persevered in, will soon bring the patient to such an ebb as to render further treatment unnecessary.

Such measures as leeches, blistering, cupping, and the like, are not only superfluous, but, I believe, in the highest degree prejudicial during these seizures. At any rate, without their exhibition I have nearly weekly seen rapid recoveries from the completest hemiplegia. Under injections, castor oil, and a Pil. Col. c. Cal., in a day or two the patient's leg begins to move, and his utterance for monosyllables to return. Later, the movements of the arm commence, and the memory, at first in abeyance, becomes sufficient to enable him to recognise and correctly to name those around him. Day by day the amelioration proceeds; and I have frequently seen a person, hemiplegic for the first time a week previously, again walking, and with his former gait, in the infirmary. Usually, however, the amendment is somewhat slower. A fortnight or three weeks may elapse before the patient quite regains his former mobility. During this time, all that is required is simply to watch, and gently to sustain the peristaltic action of the intestines.

It sometimes happens that the restored hemiplegic relapses, and has a succession of seizures, from each of which he recovers more and more imperfectly, until at length a seizure ensues, accompanied not by hemiplegia, but by complete motionless coma, and death soon follows.

It has often been noticed that a paralytic, depressed, morose, or with the low type of delusion, after a hemiplegic attack, becomes more cheerful, better tempered, and less afflicted mentally. The memory improves, the habits become less stationary, and the gait less feeble.

Generally, however, it cannot be doubted that the convalescence of each succeeding seizure finds the paralytic in a worse, though not a much worse predicament than that in which he had previously been. During the period of the seizure, a paralytic, hitherto quiet, frequently becomes restless, irritable, and incoherently talkative, particularly during the early part of the night.

From this sketch of the hemiplegia of general paralysis, it is sufficiently evident that it is a very different thing from hemiplegia, the consequence of a clot in, or of local degeneration of, the cerebrum or cerebellum. The contrast between a disorder susceptible of an easy and speedy cure, and another impracticable, tardy of amendment, and often irremediable—however many similar symptoms they may present—need scarcely be suggested. The simple remedies, facile of success in the seizures of general paralysis, are useless in those of ordinary encephalic hemiplegia. The mercurial course, the local remedies addressed to the head—which are found or considered to be of such importance in the treatment of the latter malady—are the sure means not of cure, but of further damage to the already sufficiently reduced general paralytic.

In general paralytics, who have many seizures, the hemiplegia is not always on the same side. This, as far as I know, is never observed in ordinary hemiplegics, who indeed, from the severity of their malady, are incapable of surviving *many* seizures. The grinding of the teeth, the absence of the distorted mouth, of stertor and of puffing of the lips, and the occasional presence of convulsion, likewise form a means of diagnosis. The absence of the shriek, the feebleness of the convulsion (if any), the unbitten tongue, and the presence of hemiplegia, distinguish these seizures from true epilepsy. There is indeed one rare and extraordinary malady, which might possibly be mistaken for this form of hemiplegia—hysterical paralysis.

An insane woman, by turns depressed and nymphomanic, when in the former state, on four different occasions in as many months, had unmistakeable and *unfeigned* hemiplegia sinistra. The left leg was completely powerless, and dragged after her; anæsthesia of the left

arm and leg, which were cold and mottled white and a
livid-scarlet, was nearly complete. In a couple of days
after each attack the paralysis had entirely disappeared.
A purgative, a shower-bath, and a little judicious raillery
(an excellent hysterical remedy, though sometimes inap-
plicable in private practice), were the remedies employed.
The sex of the patient, the hysterical history (which,
however, is not always to be had), and still more her
hysterical aspect, the absence of all premonitory paralytic
symptoms, whether physical or psychical, added to the
extreme rarity of the malady, render its confusion with
the hemiplegia of general paralysis, to say the least of
it, difficult. The tongue of the hysterical hemiplegic is
by no means paralyzed; on the contrary, on the eternal
subject of her own woes and maladies it is even incon-
veniently glib.

Before I close this part of the subject, I may mention
the occasional occurrence of catalepsy in connexion with
general paralysis. A paralytic, with large delusions
and markedly dilated left pupil, was admitted on the
6th of May, 1853, and discharged on the 31st of
August of the same year, all his delusions having completely disappeared. Any person, unacquainted with
the disease, would have scouted the idea of his being a
paralytic. After his removal, he many times called at
the asylum to express his gratitude, and to laugh over
his former delusions. On the 21st of November, 1853,
he returned as a patient by his own desire, with quite a
different set of delusions. He was now depressed and
apprehensive, imagining he was accused of impossible
crimes and pursued by the police. He cowered in
corners, and concealed himself behind doors. The

sound of the court-bell filled him with horror and trepidation. On the sixth day he became heavy, and was got to bed with difficulty. Half an hour afterwards he was completely comatose and motionless; the pulse was scarcely perceptible, and could not be counted. A salt injection having been given, he was placed on the night-stool, and then it was at once discovered he was cataleptic. His limbs remained exactly as the attendant left them; his figure, without support, was as erect as a statue. The legs and arms were put in positions the least convenient, and the most opposed to gravity: thus, the legs were extended straight from the hips, and the arms at right angles to the thorax. In this singular state and posture he remained a quarter of an hour, when suddenly the enema operated, and the utensil was filled with an immense number of hard fæcal lumps. The pulse on the instant rose, the rigid limbs fell, and the statue vanished. In twelve hours he was sensible and understood questions. In thirty-six hours he was walking about as usual. After three or four days he became feebler, and the weather being severe, he was kept in bed. Getting emaciated, with restless nights and heavy days, and taking food reluctantly, he gradually sank and died of paralytic exhaustion on the 3d of January, 1854 ; forty-three days after his second, and eight months after his first admission.

The third class of seizure is that in which a *recognised* paralytic is suddenly found to be stupid and bewildered, the memory nearly destroyed, the gait very feeble and tottery, the tongue and lips very tremulous, and the utterance more halting and imperfect than before. The persons, in whom this modified seizure is chiefly observed, are quiet and tractable paralytics, whose delusions, though sufficiently evident, are neither marked nor inconvenient. They are those whose arteries are rigid, whose pupils are contracted, irregular, and sluggish; the skin of whose faces resembles tinted parchment, and which is deeply indented with hard fixed lines. They are usually of advanced years, or at least over fifty. These seizures are of much more frequent occurrence in severe than in genial weather. They sometimes happen in the course of paralytic mania. A maniacal and intensely excited paralytic becomes suddenly much quieter. This welcome change, however, is evidently owing, not to an improved mental condition, but to physical inability to make as much noise, and to be as restless and destructive as heretofore. The voluble noisy incoherence sinks into low, half-formed muttering, for the tongue is semiparalysed; the restlessness and jactitation are less, for the limbs are tremulous, and their mobility abridged. The destructive propensities disappear, for the paralytic lacks power to tear. This slight seizure is sometimes the only approach to a fit, which the patient, whether excited or tranquil, has. It is none the less, however, in many instances, the harbinger of death. The patient, having in a day or two recovered from the more palpable symptoms, becomes restless, and from his greatly amended condition, is permitted to leave his bed. He wanders about purposeless, and not unfrequently bronchitis attacks him, especially during severe weather. This pulmonary affection, though slight and perfectly curable in a person of previous average health, rapidly tells on the feeble paralytic. The chest becomes suddenly oppressed, the breathing noisy and difficult, the mucous rattle in the larger bronchi painfully distinct, the lips and face livid, and the ideas more wandering; in short, all the symptoms of the circulation of venous blood, and of suffocative pulmonary obstruction, are but too evident. The paralysis of the auxiliary pectoral muscles is sufficiently shown by the nearly motionless thorax and neck, while the abdominal walls heave from the attempts of the diaphragm, by increasing the vertical diameter of the breathing area, to compensate for the diminution of the transverse. This nearly invariably fatal complication might be not improperly designated " Paralytic Bronchitis." These slight seizures often precede more marked paralysis. An insane person, who, in the course of months, may have on several occasions become for a short time tottering in gait, halting in utterance, and very stupid and bewildered, is suddenly seized with complete hemiplegia, which has all the characteristics and significance of what I have lately described as the second class of paralytic seizures.

This concludes what I have to say of the physical symptoms of General Paralysis.

CHAPTER III.

STATISTICS OF GENERAL PARALYSIS.

UNDER the head of the Statistics of General Paralysis, I propose to investigate three questions.

First. The proportion of general paralytics to be assigned to each sex.

Secondly. The age at which the disease is usually observed.

Thirdly. The duration of the disease.

And first, of the proportion of general paralytics to be assigned to either sex. The disease, from the date of its discovery, has been observed more frequently in men than in women; and to this cause is mainly due the greater number of deaths among the male patients, in those institutions for the treatment of insanity, into which all classes of patients, curable or incurable, are admitted. This disparity has, I believe, been much overstated, women having been thought to be far more rarely its subjects than turns out to be the case. The oversight, there can be little doubt, has occurred in consequence of the prevalent notion that general paralysis is always, or nearly always, associated with grand delusion; hence a large number of cases in both sexes, but especially among women, has been overlooked. The coincidence of grand delusion and general paralysis, so far from being invariable or nearly so, is not, according to my experience, observed in the majority of instances. Thus in 135 examples, which are *all* the cases occurring in my own practice of the mental condition of which I have notes, only 27 had pure unmixed magnificence of delusion, and 34 had mixed or alternating grand and depressed fancies; while in 55 instances the general type of the delusions was melancholic; and in 17 there were no delusions at all, or even any affection of the spirits.

	Males.	Females.	Total.
Elated, and the subjects of grand delusions .	22	5	27
Depressed, and the subject of melancholic delusions	36	21	57
The subjects of mixed or alternating delusions	20	14	34
Demented, and without delusion . . .	12	5	17
Total	90	45	135

The whole number of cases I have watched, and of which I have any record, is 147; of these, 96 were men, and 51 women. The disease is therefore about twice as frequent in men as in women. Of these 147 persons, 62 males and 23 females were married, 10 males and 14 females widowed, and 24 males and 14 females single. 105 patients, 67 males and 38 females, had, previous to admission, resided in towns (principally in London and Brighton); and 42 patients, 29 males and 13 females, came from rural districts. 44 (33 males and 11 females,) were private patients; and 103 (63 males and 40 females) were parochial or county patients. Most of the patients chargeable to parishes or counties were really not paupers, or at least they had only just become so by reason of their mental affliction.

THE AGE AT WHICH GENERAL PARALYSIS is usually observed is, from the care with which asylum case-books are kept, easily determinable; and perhaps it is not too much to say, that in no disease is the epoch of the greatest frequency more regular, and in few is the sexual proportion (that of 2 to 1) so nearly maintained throughout its whole career.

The appended tabular statement shows at a glance all I have been able to learn regarding the periods of the disease in either sex.

Years of Age	Males.	Females.	Total.	Absolute sexual per-centage, obtained by comparing male and female cases of each period, with the total cases of their own sex only.		Relative sexual per-centage, obtained by comparing in each period the male and female cases, with the total number of cases irrespective of sex.		General per-centage irrespective of sex.
				Male.	Female.	Male.	Female.	Total.
Between 20 and 30	6	4	10	6·25	7·843	4·081	2·720	6·802
„ 30 „ 40	36	17	53	37·50	33·338	24·489	11·564	36·054
„ 40 „ 50	30	15	45	31·25	29·411	20·408	10·204	30·612
„ 50 „ 60	18	8	26	18·75	15·686	12·244	5·442	17·687
Over 60	6	7	13	6·25	13·725	4·081	4·761	8·843
	96	51	147	100·	100·	65·303	34·691	100·

(Relative sexual per-centage totals: 65·303 + 34·691 = 100·)

From a perusal of these figures, it appears that the period of the greatest frequency in both sexes is the decade between thirty and forty, the succeeding decade, however, nearly equalling it, the respective decennial percentages being 37·5 and 31·25 for males, and 33· and 29·4 for females. For all practical purposes, then, it may be stated that the vicenniad between thirty and fifty is in both sexes the especial epoch of general paralysis, 66·6, or exactly two thirds of all the cases having occurred during those twenty years of middle life. On further examining the age of general paralytics, I have found that during the period between thirty-three and forty-five, the influences at work for the production of the malady are most active, 48 of the 96 cases in men, and 22 of the 51 female cases, having occurred during those twelve years, the per-centage for which term (61·224) is nearly equal to that (66·6) for the whole vicenniad between thirty and fifty.

The sudden accession of the malady after thirty, and its somewhat less abrupt decline after fifty, are very remarkable, and seem clearly to indicate the bearing which the trials of that eventful period of nearly every one's life have in its production. But no period of human existence—youth, early manhood, and extreme old age excepted—can claim immunity from this fell disease, its earliest and its eldest victims being respectively twenty-four and seventy-six years of age.

The proportion between the sexes (two to one) is tolerably equally maintained in the first four decades, while in the fifth (that over sixty) the disease is observed more frequently among women than men. Of 13 cases over 60, 7 occurred among women; for this period the relative male per-centage is 6·25, the corresponding female per-centage being 13·725.

DURATION OF GENERAL PARALYSIS.

The investigation of the duration of general paralysis is a subject beset with difficulties, and very unpromising of result in the present state of our knowledge: indeed of a disease, whose first symptoms have yet to be ascertained, any inquiry regarding its duration might seem superfluous or vain.

It is in the nature of chronic diseases to have beginnings slow and insidious, and to the unawakened eye differing but little from each other, or from health. The number of chronic diseases has probably been the same from an early period of our history, though, doubtless, their intensity, fatality, and even complexion, have varied much with the social or geographical condition of their subjects. The earliest symptoms of these maladies have, by the accumulated clinical observation of ages, come to be ascertained; and modern physic, by fixing their seat and causes, enables us, before the appearance of constitutional symptoms, to predict their approach, and, if not yet to repel, at least to recognise from afar these scourges of our race.

The earliest physical symptoms of phthisis and heart-disease are now, even when hardly suspected, sought for, and, because sought in the proper place and manner, often found. These diseases, however, have been recognised as the enemies of mankind for thousands of years, yet their early recognition has only become possible within the last fifty years.

Can we, then, wonder that the early symptoms of general paralysis, whose existence, though coeval with other chronic diseases, has been recognised but forty years, should be still unknown? And without this knowledge, of what avail, it may be asked, can an inquiry into its duration be? The inquiry, however fruitless at present, may avail at least this. It may possibly draw to the subject the attention of the intelligent, and enlist the sympathies of the pains-taking. And if this volume should be fortunate enough to attract the notice of the general practitioners of the United Kingdom, the mystery of the early symptoms of general paralysis and of its duration will be speedily cleared up. To the industry and acumen of that great body I especially appeal, for it supplies the medical attendants of nine-tenths of the whole population, and exclusively those of the middle and lower classes, among both of which the great majority of paralytics is to be found. The general practitioner of England is not only the physician and surgeon of his patients, but likewise their friend, confidant, and confessor. In tribulation and reverse his patients seek his aid, for apparently trifling and nameless disorders. To these indefinite maladies, the result of mental shocks, I would particularly direct his attention, as the likely soil in which the first symptoms (whatever they may be) of general paralysis are to be found, especially in fair men between thirty-three and forty-five. The wards of a hospital will not aid us much in the investigation, though doubtless from its out-patients' room, and from dispensary practice, valuable information might be gleaned.

There is, however, one symptom, which has been observed in persons not suspected of paralysis or insanity, and in whom, as yet, no intellectual decay was evident, namely, contracted and fixed, or unsymmetrical pupils. These persons have in time become incipiently paralyzed, and because paralyzed, insane. This symptom gives us a point of departure, whence to calculate the duration of the disease. These instances are, however, so few, that no positive conclusion can be drawn from them, but that the disease is of very variable and of much longer duration than is generally supposed. The late Mr. Phillips remarked the contracted and fixed pupil of the gentleman whose case I have detailed at page 8, twelve years ago. He still lives, an active, demented paralytic.

Five or six years ago, some of the mental symptoms were observed in a surgeon, who was then, and for several subsequent years, in practice; he is now an elated, demented, and destructive paralytic, under treatment in an asylum. In another gentleman, then quite sane, from his unusual irritable and overbearing temper, and from his coincident contracted and fixed pupils, general paralysis was predicted, of which, three or four years after, he died in an asylum. There are now under my notice several persons, apparently in fair mental health, who have markedly unsymmetrical, or irregular and contracted pupils, with no iritic history. Some of these persons have near relatives insane. Their subsequent history would be desirable, and might be instructive.

The duration of the disease from the commencement of the second stage (the date of recognisable insanity) is statistically a more promising subject of inquiry, though scarcely so interesting or important as its entire length.

The period of the paralytic's residence in an asylum, from his admission to his death, with the information to be gathered from the answers to the questions in "the Statement," "Age if known on first attack," and "Duration of existing attack," enables us to form a tolerably accurate notion of the duration of the malady from the first overt insane act or idea. The calculation will be doubtless only approximative, for it would be absurd to place implicit confidence in the interested testimony of relatives, or to accept for reality the result of their varying perceptions.

In the commencement of this inquiry a difficulty has to be encountered in the frequently total ignorance of those, by whom lunatic paupers are brought to asylums, of their antecedents. This ignorance, often inexcusable in other cases, is in that of a paralytic sometimes pardonable; for a wandering lunatic and a casual to the parish whence he is sent, nothing is known of his previous history. Such vague answers as "a few weeks," "some months," are nearly as great bars to our inquiry as that frequently recurring answer "not known." Thus, vagueness or absence of information greatly reduces the number of cases whence reliable inferences can be obtained. On the other hand, a large number of the paralytics, from whose cases I have lately drawn conclusions, still live, or have been removed from the asylum (it is needless to add) uncured. This again diminishes the number of cases germane to our subject, concerning the more remarkable of which I may mention a few particulars.

A merchant captain, admitted in a state of intense mania, in 1841, æt. 47, still lives, a feeble, demented, but cheerful paralytic. (He died in the autumn of 1857, having been insane sixteen years.) A carter, admitted as a paralytic maniac, in 1849, æt. 36, survives a demented melancholic. He has been insane at least five years and a half.[1] A collier captain, admitted 1853,

---

[1] Died of convulsions, occurring in the course of a sudden accession of intense paralytic mania, having been upwards of six years insane.

æt. 68, and who had been insane four years previously, survives, a demented melancholic. He has been insane eight years. A surgeon, admitted in March, 1854, æt. 39, and who had been insane three years, died 18th May, 1854. The duration of insanity was three years and a quarter. A publican, admitted 14th January, 1851, æt. 45, and who had been insane at least a year previously, died December 5th, 1853. He was, there- fore, a recognised lunatic during four years, less a month. A pawnbroker, admitted 16th February, 1846, æt. 29, died 16th February, 1854. He was insane, and resident in the asylum, eight years exactly. A lady of fortune, admitted 28th March, 1853, æt. 70, and who had been insane at least five years, died on 11th February, 1854. The duration of insanity, therefore, was six years. A poor woman, who had been two years insane prior to admission, still lives, a feeble paralytic. Her mental symptoms have been evident upwards of four years and a half.

These instances of prolonged mental derangement coincident with general paralysis, ranging between 16 and 3 years, are clearly exceptional, as, from a perusal of the appended tabular statement, it appears that of 99 cases, whence conclusions approaching accuracy can be drawn, in only 25 was the period of known insanity above three years. The more usual periods of paralytic insanity are under 3 years; for the number of cases which, between 5 and 6 years, 4 and 5 years, and 3 and 4 years, had been respectively 3, 5, and 8, suddenly rises to 19, 20, and 35, for the periods between 2 and 3 years, 1 and 2 years, and under 12 months. It thus appears, in 74 out of 99 cases the duration of alleged mental un- soundness was, for every variety of period, from $2\frac{1}{2}$

years to 22 days, 35 per cent. occurring under a year.
The cause of the larger number of instances of brief
paralytic insanity is to be sought in the fact, that the
subjects of this malady, in these cases, were nearly exclusively persons who were received from workhouses, in
the infirmaries or lunatic wards of which they had undergone a species of treatment not peculiarly adapted
for the tranquillisation of the mind, or for the prolonga-
tion of life. Thus, of the 35 instances under a year,
28 were pauper lunatics, and only 7 (or 20 per cent.)
private patients. This disproportion gradually diminishes
as we ascend towards the longer periods; thus, of the
20 and 19 instances between 1 and 2 years, and 2 and
3 years, the number of the private patients are respectively 8 and 6, or for the particular periods 40· and
31·57 per cent.; while of the 25 prolonged cases, 11
were private patients, or 44 per cent.

Private Patients Male	Private Patients Female	Pauper Patients Male	Pauper Patients Female	Years	Months	Weeks	Still alive.	Duration of Paralytic Insanity.	Total Number of Patients.
1	—	—	—	16	—	—	—	16 years	1
—	—	2	—	9	—	—	Both still alive, but feeble	9 ,,	2
2	—	—	—	8	—	—	1 still alive, feeble	8 ,,	2
—	1	—	1	7	—	—	" ,, ,,	7 ,,	2
—	—	1	—	6	6	—	Still alive, and in fair health	} Between 6 and 7 years	2
—	—	1	—	6	—	—	—		
1	—	2	—	5	—	—	2 still alive, but feeble	5 years	3
1	—	—	1	4	6	—	Both still alive, but feeble	} Between 4 and 5 years	4
1	—	1	1	4	—	—	2 alive, feeble		
1	—	—	1	3	9	—	—		
1	—	—	—	3	6	—	—		
—	—	—	1	3	3	—	—	} Between 3 and 4 years	8
2	—	—	—	3	2	—	—		
—	—	2	—	3	—	—	Both alive, and in fair health		
1	—	2	—	2	9	—	—		
—	—	3	2	2	6	—	2 alive, but feeble	} Between 2 and 3 years	19
1	—	1	4	2	3	—	2 still alive, in fair health		
4	—	1	—	2	—	—	2 still alive, in fair health		
1	—	—	—	1	9	—	alive, but feeble		
—	1	1	1	1	8	—	—	} Between 1 and 2 years	20
—	1	1	1	1	7	—	—		
—	1	2	1	1	6	—	1 still alive, and in fair health		
4	—	4	1	Between 1 and 1	4 and 1	—	—		
—	1	—	—	—	11	—	—		
—	—	5	2	—	10	—	—		
2	—	2	—	—	8	—	—		
2	—	4	1	—	7	—	—	Under a year	3
—	—	2	1	—	6	—	—		
1	—	1	—	—	5	—	—		
—	—	4	1	—	4	—	—		
—	1	2	1	—	3	—	—		
—	—	1	—	—	—	7	—		
—	—	—	1	—	—	22 days	—		
26	6	45	22				21		9
32		67							
99									

In calculating the duration of paralytic insanity, the period of alleged alienation prior to admission has been necessarily included. In many instances the paralytic had been known to be insane for a year, or many months; but in not a few cases this period is stated to be under a month, and in some only a week. Thus of 12 cases, in 5 it is said to be three weeks, in 4, two weeks, and in 3, one week. There is little doubt that, in these and all similar cases in which the friends assert that the paralytic has only been insane a few days, he has really been of unsound mind for a much longer period. Of this unsoundness the relatives may or may not be aware, according to the acuteness or dulness of their perceptions; and if it be recognised, self-interest may make its acknowledgment inconvenient.

And I may here mention my belief, that, in all cases whatsoever of general paralysis, the duration of the mental unsoundness, even if honestly stated, is understated. The slow and stealthy advance of the dementia, the gradual approach of his endless eccentricities, whims, and fancies, and generally the unpretending character of the early physical and mental symptoms, so completely break in the near relatives of the paralytic to the oddest ideas and acts, and so entirely throw them and the medical attendant off their guard, that when actions or ideas, evidently insane, supervene, they are regarded as mere accessions of that eccentricity which has been growing on him for years. But no sooner does he commit some personally violent or discreditable act, than the scales fall from their eyes, and, however unwilling to admit his gradually increasing alienation for months or years, they are ready, and even anxious, to date it from the violent or disgraceful action.

This apathy or blindness, whether of the patient's friends or physician, is the more deplorable, as it destroys all chance of his amendment, and explains the rapidity with which death, in many instances, follows a paralytic's admission into an asylum.

CHAPTER IV.

REGARDING the causes of those physical derangements, the most prominent symptom of which is insanity, little has been ascertained with certainty; though
it is reasonably surmised that in mental phenomena their
origin is usually to be found. The ætiology of general
paralysis is perhaps less obscure than that of any other
insaniferous malady; and there can be little doubt that
to powerful impressions on the moral sense, usually as
it would seem, of a painful character, the cause of the
disease is to be traced.

To moral or intellectual sensibility, to our varying
capacity for receiving pleasure or pain from mental impressions, and to the competence of its respective emotions for the causation and perhaps the cure of disease,
but cursory allusion is commonly made by writers on
medicine. This seems the more remarkable, as if we
analyse what passes within us, even superficially, we
become conscious that a sensation of pleasure or pain
naturally attends every cerebral act, and signally every
unwonted cerebral act. Except in special cases, however,
from instinctive policy or apathy, we silence or disregard
these inevitable emotional promptings; or from their con-

stant presence we entirely overlook their existence. Of
the gratification of our instincts, and of the pain felt if
that gratification be prevented or even delayed, it is unnecessary to speak; nor need I but glance at the pleasure
or pain derivable from the stimulation of the ganglia of
special sense by their appropriate irritants. The inhala-
tion of a delicious perfume, the sight of a beautiful colour,
the hearing of a pure tone, and the taste of an exquisite
dish or delicate wine, impart pleasures purely sensuous.
A nauseous taste, an offensive odour, a discordant sound,
or an ugly colour, gives unmistakeable sensuous pain.
The perception necessary for the appreciation of the arts
is of a mixed character, partaking of the sensuous and
intellectual. The works of the painter, the sculptor, or
the composer, excite in us, according to their subject or
execution, lively emotions of pleasure or pain. But in
a man, worthy of the name, the keenest of these sensations is derived from intellectual or moral impressions.
To witness, to read or hear of a noble action, to seize or
reflect on a happy idea, to master a difficult subject, are
sources of pleasure in comparison with which most others
are, or should appear, insignificant. Nor is that pain
slight which is caused by the base actions or the gro-
velling ideas of others, or with which we think of their
ingratitude or depravity. If pleasure or pain can be
thus excited by the mere contemplation of moral actions;
if, spectators of the stage of life, abstract goodness or
badness so gladdens or distresses us, how much keener
becomes our emotion, when we appear as actors in the
drama, and are deeply interested in the catastrophe.
Thus all operations commencing in or conducted by the
nervous system, from the lowest to the highest, from
mere instinct, from the perceptions of pure sense,
through the connecting link of the sensuo-intellectual to

the highest mental and moral acts, are accompanied by pleasurable or painful emotions.

The vivacity of the moral is like that of the special senses, different in different persons, or rather in no two persons are any of these exactly similar. Tolerance of physical pain varies with the individual; what is endured by one man without a murmur or grimace, produces in another frantic cries and gestures. That this difference is not the result invariably of superior fortitude, is sufficiently proved by the high courage and power of bearing which, except of physical pain, distinguishes many of these persons. Some of the nationalities, which contribute to our hybrid population, might be mentioned as illustrative of this position. A few persons are distinguished by the fineness of their taste, and to that peculiarity owe their fortunes. A tea, an opium, or a wine taster, must have received from nature superior gustative power, which doubtless can be greatly improved by education and practice. The disgust which stenches, and the delight which perfumes inspire in some persons, are well known; to others they appear equally indifferent. The power of discriminating the most delicate varieties of hue and tone are well-known and valuable faculties; nor are instances of colour-blindness and music-deafness uncommon. The power of tact is at least as capricious as any other of the special senses. In any single person, in proportion to the dulness or acuteness of the sensuous perception, will be of course the resulting sensation of pleasure or pain; but in any two persons, a perception, equally clear to either, will not cause the evolution of the same amount of these sensations, which indeed will be entirely regulated by the sensuous sensibility of the individual. Similarly vary the perceptions and susceptibility of the moral sense. One person views with horror, and is therefore pained by what another regards as nearly venial, and to which, therefore, he is indifferent. The moral view of a thing which strikes one man as peculiarly just, and which, therefore, fills him with pleasure, appears to his neighbour a distortion and as bordering on nonsense or cant: and of two persons taking precisely the same view of any moral act or idea, it will not, therefore, be true that each necessarily experiences the same degree of pleasure or pain. To early associations or prejudices, to education and to habit, much of this variety is to be ascribed; but as much at least to the natural vivacity or obtuseness of moral perceptions, and to the individual's peculiar endowment as regards moral sensibility.

As the acuteness of sensuous perceptions varies at different periods of life, so does that of the moral sense. The nicety of tact, taste, sight, smell, and hearing, probably improves till twenty-five, remains stationary till forty-five, and thence declines, *pari passu*, with advancing years. In boyhood, though the perceptions of sensuous pleasure and pain are of the keenest, moral sensibility is hardly awakened. The loss of position, or of parents, their misfortunes, or disgrace, do not acutely affect the young or even the adolescent. From twenty-five to forty-five, all these are more poignantly felt; and many a man of sixty defies the finger of scorn or the hoot of malevolence, at which, at thirty-five, he would have winced; and braves the storm of misfortune or of slander, under which at the same age he would have succumbed. Though the old man's experience may have taught him to bear without flinching, perhaps to disregard, the world's opinion, his diminished sensibility renders the teaching of his experience less necessary.

On persons of a fine moral sensibility, unmerited disgrace or unkindness, the misfortunes of their relatives, the knowledge of their own shortcomings, baseness, or crimes, weighs heavily. Though a mind with an average moral sensibility is to be regarded as psychically normal, and with a finer sensitiveness as gifted, yet an exquisite susceptibility of the moral sense is nearly as great a misfortune as can happen to its subject. Life is to him nothing but a long ecstacy, an alternation of rapture and despair, in which, from the constitution of society as it at present exists, misery is likely to be largely in the ascendant. This moral hyperæsthesia, if contained in a feeble body (as it usually is), and occurring in a person who has to make his own way in the world, is tolerably certain to be sooner or later the cause of severe physical, and probably of cerebral disease.

Having thus given a brief account of moral sensibility, I have now to state on what grounds is based the assertion, that an acutely painful impression on it is the usual cause of general paralysis. The only means I have of ascertaining the ascribed causes of *all* the cases is from the " statement " of the order on which the paralyzed lunatic is admitted into an asylum. Of the history of many I am accurately informed ; to that of the remainder the " statement " is my sole guide. The nearly invariably ascribed cause (when any is given), whether mentioned in the statement or received orally from the patient's friends, is some form of painful moral shock. Though the popular account of the causation of anything medical is to be received with the greatest caution, yet to a uniformity of ascribed origin it is impossible to deny the merit of approximative accuracy. The explanation of the unusual popular correctness in the ætiology of general paralysis seems to lay in the salient nature of the causes. A man who has witnessed a frightful accident, and hears in a few days that some of the victims are dead, will probably ascribe the fatal result to the right cause. A person, who hears of his neighbour's domestic affliction and sees his mental anguish, recognises in it the cause of his subsequent madness. The unhappy bankrupt's friends, seeing how he takes his misfortune to heart, fear for his sanity, and not without reason.

In the paralytic's history there is a recent event which stands out from his life as its most startling, and usually as its most painful feature.

With these prefatory remarks, I will give a list of the ascribed origin of all the cases in which a history was to be had. The moral causes will form a melancholy catalogue of misery and disaster. In fifty-two instances the disease was thus accounted for:

Family anxiety, loss of position, death of relative.
Remorse from profligacy.
Loss of several children from typhus fever.
Death of daughter.
Sister's madness.
Contemplation of the misery and poverty of her parents and relatives.
Bankruptcy, a publican.
Grief at transportation of husband.
Disappointment in marriage.
Grief at her husband's profligacy.
Disappointment in marriage.

Bankruptcy, a butcher.
Commercial ruin, a German merchant.
Ditto.
Commercial ruin, a stockbroker.
Commercial ruin, a sharebroker.
Husband's death.
Brother's death.
Remorse from profligacy.
Family troubles and commercial disaster.
Depression of trade.
Loss of livelihood and protracted suffering from chronic rheumatism.

Wife's death.

Bankruptcy, a grocer.

Bankruptcy, a farmer.

Bankruptcy, a publican.

Overwrought by long and continued teaching.

Destitution.[1]

Wife's insanity.

Disappointment.

Domestic anxiety and commercial disaster.

Anxiety of business and family trouble.

Want.[1]

Grief at loss of wife.

Grief at slander on wife.

Death of brothers and children; loss of position and business.

Loss of livelihood and means of keeping his family, in consequence of broken leg.

Sudden loss of two good situations.

Commercial disaster.

Ditto.

Ingratitude and violence of son.

Remorse from profligacy.

Loss of position from disreputable marriage.

Ditto.

Professional disappointment.

Unhappy and unsuitable marriage.

Commercial anxiety.

Loss of daughter.

Remorse for crimes; shame at their punishment.

Loss of position; commercial disaster.

Death of son.

Anxiety in consequence of slanderous accusation.

Ten cases are attributed to intemperance; and in 6 instances a symptom of the disease, epileptiform seizures, was mistaken for its cause. Four cases are

---

[1] Destitution though, primâ facie, exclusively a physical, is really in a far intenser degree a moral cause of disease. It is, indeed, usually the catastrophe of a long and hard fought struggle against misfortune, often against hope. It may be the last trial of honest, but impatiently borne poverty, or the last step in a descent from a reputable rank in life. In the latter case especially, and in a sensitive person, it implies nearly any conceivable amount of protracted moral pain.

ascribed to cranial injury, and 5 respectively to "Fever," "Exposure to heat and cold," "Exposure during harvest," lactation and debauchery. Concerning the causes of the remaining 70 cases nothing is known, either because there was no assignable cause, or because, from the patient being a casual or a wanderer, his previous history in the place whence he was sent to the asylum was unknown. It thus appears that in 52 of the 77 cases in which causes were given, the insanity of the paralytic was ascribed to painful mental shocks. This is the same thing as saying that these shocks were the cause of the general paralysis; for, although the informants were not aware of the patients' condition, the latter were insane, simply because they were incipiently paralysed. The 10 cases, which are attributed to intemperance, will strike those who seem inclined to ascribe every ill that flesh is heir to, to the abuse of alcoholic drinks, as too few. However willing to admit drunkenness as a frequent source of physical disease, I very much doubt the truth of the reiterated assertion, that it is often the immediate cause of insanity, and still more of general paralysis. It is more than probable that, in the 10 cases above mentioned, the mind was already giving way, when the incipient paralytic gave way to liquor, and that he flew to the alcoholic consoler to escape from that overwhelming care in which is to be sought the true cause of his malady. That the disease is hastened by intemperance is likely; but inasmuch as the very characteristic psychical symptoms, the result of intemperance, are entirely wanting in general paralysis, drunkenness cannot be conceded as a primary, though it is doubtless, in some cases, a powerful auxiliary cause.

In 6 cases, the paralytic seizures being mistaken by

medical men for epilepsy, the insanity was ascribed to that disease. The causes of the 4 cases attributed to local injury are, I believe, wrongly given. The incipient dementia of the patient, his forgetfulness and preoccupation, render him peculiarly liable to accidents; and his irritable vehemence is a fruitful source of violence, which, usually commencing with himself, is sometimes returned with interest by the attacked party. Two of these paralytics received severe blows on the head during quarrels, the third was thrown from his horse, which for several months previously he had taken to ride with unusual impetuosity. The fourth case is not so easy to analyse. An able surgeon, who had been unsuccessful in his professional career, in 1851 was stunned in a railway accident. He had during the following month trifling paralytic symptoms, confined to the left side of the face. Eighteen months from the date of the accident his boisterous manner and absence of mind were remarked: nine months subsequently he was recognised as insane. He died of apoplexy, having been insane at least two years and a quarter. It is difficult to ascertain whether pain at his failure in life, which he felt acutely, or the railway accident, the more contributed to the causation of his paralytic insanity. It is probable that the accident, unaided by the previous moral shock, would have been insufficient for the production of the disease, though doubtless competent to hasten its development.[1]

Regarding the cases, to the causes of which the immediate relatives can or will give no clue, it may be

---

[1] Many months after this patient's death, I for the first time saw his father, who informed me that *three years before* the railway accident his son had had a slight and evanescent attack of paralysis.

said that this large group militates strongly against the assertion that general paralysis usually originates in acutely painful emotions. The validity of this objection I cannot admit. Your informant is the near relative of the paralytic, and is implicated, perhaps not very creditably, in the production of the moral anguish which is the real cause of the malady. Will a daughter or wife, to satisfy the cravings of the ætiologist, acknowledge her own neglect or dishonour; or will a husband or a son admit his own misconduct or ingratitude? But it is highly probable that, in some cases at least, the relatives are really unaware of any painful moral impression. The diffident and reserved brood over their cares and apprehensions, and hug them to their own destruction, Without the vent of confidence, their wretchedness ferments, and expanding in its usually feeble inclosing case, soon bursts and shatters it. The paralytic and his friends may be persons of totally different moral impressibility. Words and actions, which to him are acutely painful, in them excite no emotion. The two persons see nothing from the same moral point of view. Hence he shuns their confidence, and hides his anxiety rather than reveal it to be ridiculed. The incessant strife of strongly opposed moral natures is wearing, and the weaker, after an obstinate, and to him exhausting conflict, gives way. Yet the unintentional antagonist does not see, and indeed is incapable of comprehending the cause of the spectacle before him. The victim is extremely sensitive, he is morally thin-skinned; sanguine perhaps, and greatly depressed by reverse, urged on by moral temerity, but endowed with only feeble fortitude. The domestic opponent is by nature calm, impassive, and insusceptible, his enthusiasm difficult to kindle, his head to convince. Of a hard, but not a bad disposition, he cannot understand the fine feelings, as he calls them, of his relative; unimpressible or apathetic, he despises his woes as imaginary or affected. It is evident that in this sad conflict of opposite temperaments both are wrong. The emotions of the one, whether of pleasure or pain, are causelessly acute and too easily called forth; those of the other too feeble and too difficult of evolution. And it is often from the mental survivor of this unrecognised struggle that the psychologist receives the history of the case. Of the existence of the struggle he is not aware, so he tells you, and honestly, that he knows of no cause for his friend's insanity.

The complexion, the age, the social condition, the habitat, and the sex of the majority of general paralytics, all favour the idea that moral agony is the cause of the disease.

The nearly universal fair complexion of its victims would seem to indicate that the mental collapse of the sanguine temperament is frequently so complete as to overturn the reason. The reaction from elated self-reliant confidence to blank despair, the prostration of the latter condition being in an inverse proportion to the elevation of the former, is so overwhelming as to produce a molecular or organic change in that portion of the encephalon which presides over and directs the spirits, which is the organ in which all sensations of pleasure or pain take place. It is, therefore, because the blue-eyed and fair-complexioned are too sanguine and too susceptible, because their exulting confidence sometimes hurries them into difficulties, in consequence of which their morbid sensibility becomes deeply wounded, that they are by far the most frequent victims of general paralysis.

Of 147 cases, 100 had blue, gray, or light hazel eyes; 11 had dark eyes, and of 36 the colour of the iris is not recorded.

	Males.	Females.	Total.
Light eyes	65	35	100
Dark eyes	6	5	11
Colour not recorded	25	11	36
Total	96	51	147

The epoch of general paralysis, its greater frequency between thirty and fifty in both sexes, and especially between thirty-three and forty-five in men, is to my mind strongly confirmatory of its supposed moral origin. Between twenty and thirty usually happen those events which settle our fate for life. The professional man completes his education, and launches into practice; the merchant enters on his commercial career; and the tradesman opens his shop. All three marry. The result of these steps is not at once apparent. For their development, whether happy or disastrous, ten or fifteen years are perhaps required. In ten years from his outset the lawyer or surgeon has become tolerably sure what his future prospects will be. His small capital is either frittered away, or is paying him magnificent interest. A prosperous future, or the darkening vista of indigence, opens before him. The young merchant or manufacturer, with the unimpaired energy and talent of thirty-five, is on the road to a plum or an almshouse.

The spirited tradesman exhausts all the modern arts of the counter, in the hope of competence and position following his exertions. But a keen competition often beats him; and he is as frequently foiled by his own excessive cleverness, by carrying too far, even for this not very squeamish age, the tricks and craft of his trade.

It is from the aspiring middle class, and from the more energetic of its next lower grade—from those who, dependent on neither wealth nor interest, have to win their way unaided in the world—that the numerous victims of general paralysis are recruited. By thirty-five or forty, that is, ten or fifteen years after their launch into life, disaster, if misfortune is to be their lot, overtakes them. By this time the germ of unsuccess has had time to shoot. Inaptitude for their calling, from want of talent, temper or tact, unbusiness-like habits, indolence or timidity, intemperance, speculation, or want of thrift,—any of these may be the rock on which they split; or some of those inevitable and un-looked-for mischances, incidental to the early struggles of the commercial or the professional career, may surprise them. The identity of the epoch of these calamities, and of the greatest frequency of general paralysis, is not mere coincidence. It is precisely because the struggling merchant, trader, mechanic, or professional man, is stricken down by self-produced or accidental disaster, at an age when his moral sensibility is at its height, that he is, in the very prime of life, so common a martyr to the disease.

The ten or fifteen years following the wedding-day are the most trying of married life. The birth of children in quick succession, and the necessary efforts for their maintenance and education are, among the needy but conscientious of the middle and lower classes, no mean sources of care and anxiety. The parents' passions are still high, and their susceptibility may be keen. In a well-assorted marriage this conjunction is fortunate, it is a cause of present and an earnest of future happiness; in an unsuitable one, it can hardly be other than the fertile source of misery, and perhaps of struggle against temptation, not always resistible. Beside the trials of unfortunate or unholy wedlock, there are some even more severe, incidental and indeed in proportion to its full and hallowed fruition. The more perfect the union the more overwhelming will be the shock of its sudden disruption, and the closer the clinging of parental love the intenser will be the agony of its severance. What more genuine or more enduring sorrow is there than that which mourns a loved young wife or only child, or than attends the supervention of widowhood, poverty-stricken perhaps, or otherwise calamitous? It would seem, therefore, if the moral wear and tear of early married life has not been not overstated, that a preponderance of married general paralytics is to be expected. The statistics of the disease confirm this view. Of 147 general paralytics, 85 were married, 24 widowed, and 38 single.

	Males.	Females.	Total.	
Married	62	23	85	} 109
Widowed	10	14	24	
Single	24	14	38	
Total	96	51	147	

Thus 109, or 74·1 per cent. of all the cases were or had been married.

The favorite habitat of the disease is strongly corroborative of its moral origin. The great majority of general paralytics, who are admitted into asylums, have been resident in large towns. From London and Brighton the worst cases, that have come under my notice, have been sent.

To London, the cloaca gentium, itself the seat of reckless speculation and daring profligacy, come from every other quarter the wretched and the vile to hide themselves from infamy or care; and the moral atmosphere of watering-places of rapid growth is of the lowest, their commercial condition of the most unsound.

The anguish or remorse, which eventually overtakes persons afflicted by a moral hyperæsthesia, and who, whether tempters or victims, feel self-degraded by debauchery and social crime, will always be most rife in capitals and large towns. In cities there is always more vice, and, therefore, more mental misery, because they possess many temptations to suggest, many incentives to and opportunities for, the gratification of the passions, which are wanting in rural districts.

The domestic distress, which the sudden slackness of an important branch of manufacture, or which the stoppage of a large commercial house, always entails on the principals, but especially on their clerks and workmen, and the periodical collapse of many trades, as carpenters, bricklayers, &c., in winter, are always more keenly felt in towns; where, in fact, the larger number of workmen and of artisans reside. The less regular life of the town workman renders him, likewise, a more easy prey to cerebral as to ordinary physical disease.

Accordingly, we find that of 147 paralytics, 105 were admitted from towns, and only 42 from rural districts.

	Males.	Females.	Total.	Per-centage.
Sent from Towns	67	38	105	71·42
Sent from Rural Districts . .	29	13	42	28·57
Total	96	51	147	100·

The preponderance of male paralytics is a fact of great significance, and is strongly corroborative of the moral origin of the disease.

Female tolerance of physical pain is too well known a fact to require any present notice, nor can any candid observer deny woman's superior, though not always silent, endurance of moral pain. Accordingly, of the victims of general paralysis only one third are women; and why is it so? It is not because the moral perception of women is dull, for I believe their discrimination of right and wrong approaches nearer intuition than men's; it is not because they are less sensitive, for I believe they feel more acutely. It is that despite their quick moral perception and lively sensibility, notwithstanding the greater frequency of the severest tests of their patience, their superior fortitude carries them through trials and over difficulties which would have bowed to the earth the physically stronger, and perhaps more intellectual sex. One of the most convincing proofs of feminine endurance is the very few cases of insanity that happen among the unfortunates, whose only means of living is prostitution. The feeling of self-degradation, the contempt of the world, the remembrance of their former innocence, their isolation and occasional physical wretchedness, the result of intemperance, disease or poverty, are yet insufficient to drive them mad; though an impulse of disgust or remorse sometimes urges them to hide themselves from infamy in the suicide's grave.

The comparative immunity of women from general paralysis and their greater moral endurance, the frequency of the disease among men and their ready prostration under calamity, go far to prove that an acute susceptibility to and an intolerance of moral pain, are among the most frequent causes of the malady.

CHAPTER V.

CASES AND AUTOPSIES.

From a larger number of cerebral autopsies of general paralysis, I have selected twenty-six as fully and exactly enough reported for accurate inference. From a comparison of these reports, which are completely in unison with my reminiscences of other cases, I hope to be able to indicate the seat and nature of the morbid changes in the brain, to which the physical and mental symptoms of the malady are due. Each autopsy will be preceded by its case, as concisely related as perhaps it is desirable, of a long, a variable, and a comparatively unknown disease.

Case I.—J. T. O—, æt. 40, an omnibus-driver, married; admitted May 31st, 1855, from London.

A short sallow man, of small frame, emaciated, in very feeble physical condition. Skin cool; lips and hands livid; facial expression fatuous, with no play of feature. Eyes brown; pupils dilated, unequal, left rather the larger. Nostrils equal, motionless. Upper lip long, straight. Mouth very broad. Tongue large, tremulous, furred. Pulse 92, full from arterial rigidity. Gait feeble, and utterance defective.

He is not very incoherent, but semi-demented. Says he is heir to £50,000 under his uncle's will. He is reported to be very violent. Said to have been insane ten days. No known cause for his insanity. Ext. Hyoscy. Əj, o. n.[1]

June 2d.—Ext. Hyoscy. ʒss, bis die.

3d.—Has been highly excited and utterly incoherent since admission. Has very bad nights, and is usually excited in the day. To-day he is kneeling, and, in the tone and with the gestures of mental anguish, repeating the Creed. Right pupil the larger.

7th.—Has continued full of the most horrible fancies; says he has "seduced his sister," and that he is "poisoned with arsenic," &c. Ext. Hyoscy. ʒss, bis terve die.

27th.—Has continued excited and full of frightful delusions. His melancholic mania, though constant, has been of very varying intensity. When at its highest pitch, temporary seclusion in a padded room was required. When more calm, and when his delusions were less vivid, he was quite manageable at large. He is now calm. The ʒss Ext. Hyoscy. twice or thrice a day has been continued till to-day, and with the effect of tranquillising him for a few hours after its exhibition. The right pupil has been the more dilated whenever looked at, since the 3d instant. Omitte Hyoscy.

July 25th.—Melancholic delusions continue. To-day he is tranquil, and walking about the airing-court. Since admission has taken food tolerably well.

28th.—An enema salis brought away an immense quantity of small, hard, rounded scybala.

---

[1] It has been stated by some prescribers that the extract of henbane is an uncertain, often an inert, preparation. My experience of it tells me, on the contrary, that it is a remedy as certain as opium, when given in adequate doses. It produces sleep or tranquillity, never dangerous narcotism. In cases of intense cerebral excitement supervening on chronic, recurrent, acute, or paralytic mania, I have given, dosibus gradatim auctis, thousands of ʒss or Əij doses of the extract, and never with any inconvenient result. The dilatation of the pupil by ten-grain or Əj doses, even when tranquillity is not attained, proves conclusively the genuineness of the drug. The only extracts of henbane of which I have any large experience, are those prepared by the Society of Apothecaries, Blackfriars, by Herring Brothers, of Aldersgate Street, and by Mr. Morson, of Southampton Row. I have not noticed any variation in their respective articles.

30th.—Has been more tranquil; usually up and walking in the airing-court.

31st.—Very wretched in padded room. Right pupil the more irregular; both pupils contracted.

August 7th.—Since 31st has been tranquil and at large.

8th.—Frightfully excited from horrible fancies. Secluded.

9th.—Quiet from exhaustion, in bed.

11th.—Takes his food with reluctance. Right pupil markedly the larger.

15th.—Silent, but making the most eloquent gestures, indicative of fear and horror.

16th.—Takes food very sparingly; continues silent.

17th.—Up to-day; not depressed.

18th.—Walking about.

19th.—Good-humoured, very well-disposed, and grateful to his attendant.

20th.—Very apprehensive. Right pupil the larger.

24th.—In padded room, in a condition of melancholic mania.

30th.—Has been at large since the 24th. He is very incoherent and depressed. Right pupil the larger, markedly.

September 2d.—At 6½ a.m. was intensely excited, from melancholic delusions. Had Ext. Hyoscy. ʒss, since which he has been tranquil. Pupils dilated wide at noon.

3d.—Comparatively tranquil; walking about.

4th.—Has passed a frightful night in padded room. He is excited now, but not from low fancies. Ext. Hyoscy. ʒss, bis die.

9th.—Has been tranquil since the 4th. The Hyoscyamus, producing diarrhœa, has been discontinued.

10th.—In padded room. Both pupils contracted; right the larger.

15th.—Has continued tolerably tranquil.

16th.—In padded room, groaning and gesticulating horribly.

18th.—Singing all manner of nonsense; at large yesterday and to-day. He is elated, and his gestures are of the drollest.

20th.—In padded room; very depressed.

24th.—Full of all manner of droll antics.

25th.—Talking elatedly in bed.

26th.—Crying and gesticulating horribly.

27th.—Quiet.

28th.—Elated and talkative.

October 5th.—Has been usually cheerful and more calm.

6th.—Highly excited, in padded room. Ext. Hyoscy. ℥ss, statim.

8th.—Excitement continues; he is, however, at large. Ext. Hyoscy. ℥ss, bis die.

13th.—Has been tolerably tranquil till to-day. He is now howling in mental agony.

15th.—Maniacal depression continues.

19th.—Talking to himself in a melancholic strain. Right pupil markedly the larger.

21st.—Good-tempered and elated. Right pupil very slightly the larger.

31st.—Has been intensely excited since the 21st; sometimes drank his own urine, and was destructive of clothing and bedding.

November 1st.—Elated and talkative; walking about with a flower in his button-hole.

2d and 3d.—Continues in the same pleasant condition. Pupils are equal.

6th.—Restless and very feeble; in bed.

13th.—Has been highly excited since the 6th. Has a large prolapsus ani, produced by the violence of his gestures and bearing down.

15th.—Extremely feeble; quiet.

17th.—After a restless night, during which he constantly said he knew he should die soon, at $5\frac{1}{3}$ a.m. he became silent, but was still restless. He continued so till within a few minutes of his death, which took place at $7\frac{1}{2}$ a.m., and was unattended by convulsion.

Autopsy, fifty-one hours after death.—Body very emaciated. Scalp bloodless; stripped off with some difficulty. Skull of normal thickness, but of ivory-like closeness of texture. Dura mater dense. Arachnoid free from adhesions, except at the inner edge of the hemispheres, corresponding to the sagittal suture. Here the attachment was so intimate, that the pia mater was torn off in removing the dura mater. No subarachnoid or inter-convolutional serum. Surface of brain normally vascular.—*Base of brain.* Internal carotids widely patent, not atheromatous. Both middle cerebral arteries atheromatous in patches, right by far the more so; its sides flattened, but caliber increased. Vertebrals free from atheroma. Basilar markedly atheromatous, the posterior cerebral arteries also. Both corpora albicantia indistinct, of a dirty white colour, and soft. The right corpus albicans could hardly be identified. Tuber cinereum healthy. In tracing the middle cerebral artery through the fissura sylvii, the lower surface of the middle lobe, corresponding to right inferior ventricular cornu and lower part of the right thalamus, was discovered to be nearly diffluent. Pia mater did not strip off convolutions very easily. Gray matter darkish and bloodless. Puncta large, numerous, coloured, and irregularly shaped in left centrum ovale. In right centrum fewer, uncoloured, and filled with thread-like fibrinous clots. Corpus callosum normal. Fornix nearly diffluent. Commissura mollis none, or any vestige of it. Right thalamus at least a third less in size than the left, bloodless, softish, with large empty (apparently vascular) channels in its substance. Right corpus striatum similarly smaller than the left. Vessels on surface of left thalamus and corpus striatum healthy and normally numerous. None visible on the corresponding right ganglia. Medulla oblongata, pons, crura cerebri and cerebellum healthy. Radial and brachial arteries patent, with no diminution of caliber at their cut extremities.

CASE II.—Th. S——, æt. 53, married, a London mason; admitted March 11th, 1855.

A fair good-looking man, of average frame and middle height, in very feeble physical condition. Skin cool; complexion a delicate pink. Expression vacant, neither elated or depressed. Eyes gray; pupils unequal, irregular, contracted; left markedly the more irregular, its axis diverging.

Head well shaped. Tongue furred, large, and tremulous; utterance hardly intelligible. Pulse 64. Arteries rather rigid. Gait tottering. He is lame from an old injury of the left leg, which is markedly inverted.

He is quite incoherent, and his memory is greatly impaired. Talks of his large estate at Worthing. He is quiet and well conducted. His insanity is attributed to grief at the severe accident to his leg, which happened fourteen months previous to his admission, and which deprived him of the means of livelihood, and of supporting his family.

28th.—Very well disposed, cheerful, and industrious. He is physically stronger. Delusions large: talks of the £30,000 a year he fancies he has, and of his pack of hounds and park at Worthing.

May 26th.—He is much stronger physically; mentally the same. Constantly rolling the yard. Left pupil as heretofore.

October 15th.—Has been working for several months at his trade, under the guidance of the bricklayer; climbs up high ladders, carries hods of mortar, &c. Delusions continue of the same type.

January 15th, 1856.—Very cheerful and well-disposed. Delusions unchanged. Pupils as heretofore.

March 31st.—Suddenly seized with convulsed coma. Except when convulsed he is motionless. An enema salis brought away an immense quantity of small hard scybala. Deglutition in abeyance.

April 3d.—Occasional convulsion continues; coma profound. He cannot swallow.

4th.—More conscious, only semi-comatose. Right arm motionless and insensible; swallows with difficulty; convulsive twitches of face and limbs continue. Enema salis.

5th.—Convulsions have returned with increased violence. Evidently sinking.

6th.—Right arm paralysed and insensible. No responsive movement when a finger is pinched. Both legs and the left arm move freely on pinching; the movements of the latter, however, are much the less lively. Swallows with difficulty.

8th.—Died.

Autopsy.—Scalp peals off readily. Skull of normal thickness and texture. Dura mater healthy. Arachnoid adherent along the posterior half of the line corresponding to the sagittal suture. Subarachnoid and interconvolutional serum abundant. Left centrum ovale rather the smaller. Copious serum in ventricles. Left thalamus and corpus striatum the smaller. Left side of the fornix half the width of the right, and diffluent. Commissura mollis none. Arteries atheromatous in patches.

CASE III.—J. B—, æt. 41, single, a farm-labourer ; admitted February 24th, 1855.

An emaciated sallow man, of average frame and height, to the last degree feeble. Facial expression low ; face thin, cheeks hollow, malar bones prominent and high. Skin hottish. Tongue dry from incessant talking. Pulse, though full, cannot be counted, as he is so restless. Arteries markedly rigid and tortuous. He is so feeble he can scarcely walk. Pupils regular, very unequal ; right dilated wide. Utterance slightly halting.

He is always talking incoherently, and is in the highest degree destructive, morose, and violent. He has no large delusions.

He is stated to have been insane two months ; the cause is unknown. There is a history of intemperance. There are sores on both hips, over the sacrum, and on one heel. Ext. Hyoscy. Əj statim, in a pint of porter and eggs. Ext. Hyoscy. ʒss, h. s.

25th.—As it is found impossible to keep him in the infirmary, in consequence of his intense maniacal raving and restlessness, he is placed in the padded room. Ext. Hyoscy. ʒss ter die, in porter and eggs.

26th.—He is somewhat quieter, but very difficult to manage. Ext. Hyoscy. Əij, ter die.

27th.—His maniacal moroseness continues. A showerbath, of a minute's duration, had not the smallest effect in calming him. Continue the Ext. Hyoscy. Əij ter die.

28th.—Has passed the night raving. At 10 a.m. took

Ext. Hyoscy. Ʒij in porter. He is now (noon) quiet and rather drowsy; but violently refuses food. Continue ext. Ʒij ter die.

March 2d.——He is quieter; has had two tolerable nights, and takes liquid food fairly.

3d.——Continues rather noisy; he is destructive, tears blankets, &c. Bowels confined. Ol. Croton, ♏j, statim.

4th.——Bowels open, motion lumpy. Takes food reluctantly.

5th.——Refuses food and medicine; his maniacal symptoms are as intense as ever.

6th.——He is quieter, but feebler; speech more halting; takes food more freely. Continue Ext. Hyoscy. Ʒij ter die.

10th.——Has continued intensely excited since the 6th. Always morose. Right pupil always dilated wide. He gets daily feebler. The henbane has calmed him for a few hours after its exhibition.

11th.—— Sinking. Both pupils dilated wide; he squints; takes food and physic sparingly, and is still as obstinate and as ill conditioned as his failing strength permits him to be. Died at midnight.

Autopsy.——Scalp very tough, and detached with difficulty. Skull thick. Dura mater healthy. Arachnoid free from adhesions; pia mater gorged. Arteries full of blood. Pia mater pealed easily off convolutions, which were pale and bloodless. Medullary substance studded with numerous large puncta, many of which were triangular. The right corpus striatum and thalamus softened nearly to diffluence, readily broken down by a stream of water, and markedly smaller than the corresponding left ganglia, which are apparently healthy. No fluid in ventricles. Right corpus albicans, and right half of the tuber cinereum, are softish. Medulla oblongata slightly softened. Cerebral arteries atheromatous in patches, and all more or less patent. Brachial and radial patent, and full of blood. Large fibrinous clots in left ventricle. Aorta markedly atheromatous.

CASE IV.—J. C. M——, æt. 41, a shoemaker, married; admitted November 30th, 1854.

A fair man, of powerful frame, above middle height, not thin, in feeble physical condition. Skin cool; complexion a diffused unhealthy red. Facial expression vacant, unvarying, not elated or depressed; face itself fat and pendulous. Utterance very halting. Gait, a feeble roll. Upper lip long and straight. Nostrils equal, compressed, motionless. Eyes gray; pupils very sluggish, equal.

Memory gone, cannot tell how many children he has, nor their names or ages. He is not incoherent, and the spirits are equable. He has been insane nine months.

In this case there are no marked mental symptoms to record beyond those sufficiently evident on his admission. At night he was often restless and destructive, and sometimes dirty. During the whole period of his residence he had no delusions, and his spirits were unaffected. Gradually sinking, he died of exhaustion, hastened by a trifling diarrhœa, on March 22d, 1855.

Autopsy, seventy-two hours after death.—Scalp tough and adherent. Skull of average thickness. Brain of medium size. Dura mater not adherent to skull. Arachnoid extensively adherent over the upper and inner mesian edge of both hemispheres. Adhesions old and granular, here and there studded with yellow earthy matter. Pia mater not much injected. Sub-arachnoid serum copious. Convolutional neurine thin, pale, and apparently bloodless. Puncta in medullary substance normal. Ventricles distended by serum. Corpus callosum soft, especially on the right side of the raphé. Fornix very soft. The right corpus striatum decidedly the larger, and the softer to a stream of water. Thalami very small, but equal and apparently normal. Commissura mollis broken down. Crura cerebri soft to the stream. The cut arteries at the base have broadly patent orifices; their coats, though free from atheroma, are unusually thick. These vessels contain scarlet blood. Tuber cinereum healthy. Medulla oblongata is perhaps soft to the stream.

Case V.—C. C——, æt. 45, married, a bankrupt publican; admitted January 27th, 1855, from Brighton.

A fair, gray-haired man, below middle height, of small frame, in very feeble physical condition. Facial expression vacant, bewildered, wooden. Eyes gray, pupils irregular, contracted, and sluggish. Nostrils equal, motionless. Lips not tremulous. Upper lip long, straight, not quite devoid of chiselling. Tongue furred white, not large or tremulous. Utterance very imperfect. Gait tottering and straddling. Pulse 92.

He is lost and bewildered, cannot answer the simplest question properly, is taciturn, and never smiles; stationary, solitary, and apparently depressed. He is stated to have been insane two months. The attributed cause is failure in business.

The mental symptoms did not vary from those already described. On one occasion only he had a delusion of a melancholic character.

Gradually sinking, he died of exhaustion of nervous power, hastened by a trifling diarrhœa, on March 17th, 1855.

Autopsy.—Skull thin. Dura mater healthy. Arachnoid normal. Pia mater congested, does not strip easily off convolutions, some of the surface of which is torn off with it. Cortex thin, of a pale buff-gray colour, and nearly exsanguine. Medullary neurine marked with numerous livid triangular puncta. Corpus callosum soft. Fornix very soft, easily broken down by a stream of water. Corpora striata and optic thalami small, else normal. Corpora albicantia very soft, and readily broken down by the stream. Cerebellum and medulla oblongata perhaps softened slightly. From the brain dribbled several ounces of darkish arterial blood. Arteries full of livid-red blood. Internal carotids quite patent. All the cerebral arteries more or less patent; a conspicuous speck of atheroma at the confluence of vertebrals. Radial and brachial patent uncontractile tubes of uniform caliber.

Case VI.—T. E——, æt. 26, married, formerly a horse-breaker; convicted of felony, October 29th, 1855; admitted December 1st, 1855. A criminal lunatic from Lewes Gaol.

A powerfully-built man of middle height, emaciated, in very feeble physical condition. Skin natural. Facial expression low, morose, and cunning. Eyes gray; pupils markedly unequal; the right contracted and nearly insensible, the left of normal size and sensitiveness. Alæ nasi conspicuously contracted at the superior edge of the cartilages. Upper lip long, straight, unchiselled; mouth very broad. Tongue large, livid, clean, not tremulous. Pulse 84, full. Utterance and gait not affected. He is bruised all over.

He is intensely excited, and utterly incoherent; morose and with no large delusion. He is to the last degree destructive; has torn up in the night two blankets, two rugs, a night-shirt, and a pillow-case. (Case taken on December 2d.)

Two days after his conviction for felony he was recognised as insane. From October 31st he has been uniformly but increasingly morose, savage, and destructive. A brother and sister of his mother were insane; one of them an epileptic. Ext. Hyoscy. Əj, bis die.

December 3d.—Right pupil slightly larger than yesterday, the left fully dilated by the henbane. He continues very savage, and is constantly threatening in his demeanour and language, talks of kicking, biting, &c. Ext. Hyoscy. ₃ss, bis die.

4th.—Has passed a frightful night in a single room.

5th.—Has torn up, during the night, two blankets and a sheet. Expression morose, language menacing. Visited by his wife, whom, pretending to embrace, he attacked. Ext. Hyoscy. ₃ss, ter die.

7th.—Intensely excited, morose, dirty, and destructive. Omit Hyoscy. Liq. Opii, ₃ss, ter die.[1]

---

[1] Liq. Opii, whenever mentioned in this volume, is an aqueous solution of crude opium, ₃j of which contains so much of the active principles of Əss of the drug as are soluble in *distilled water*, acidulated with citric acid. It is therefore a solution of citrate of morphia, codeia, and of the other

9th.—He is rapidly emaciating under the intense excitement, which continues unabated. Continue opium.

12th.—The opium being found of no avail in calming him, was left off to-day. To resume Ext. Hyoscy. ʒss, bis die.

14th.—No mental improvement. In bed, physically very feeble; takes food reluctantly.

15th.—At 11 a.m., although evidently dying, he picked, very dexterously, two people's pockets. Died at 7.45 p.m. of exhaustion. The relative condition of the pupils never varied from that observed on admission.

Autopsy, sixteen hours after death.—Scalp tough, nearly bloodless. Skull thick anteriorly; diploe congested. Cranial cavity not large, much smaller anteriorly than behind. Temporal muscles not large. Half an inch to the right of the junction of the sagittal and coronal suture, and in the frontal bone, was a deep, irregular, diaphanous pit, an inch broad by nearly an inch in length; there was no similar depression on the left side. Dura mater healthy. Arachnoid adherent along mesian longitudinal line of both hemispheres. Adhesions old, whitish, granular. Surface vessels gorged, dark purple. Sub-arachnoid serum trifling. Pia mater peals off readily, very congested, of a dull livid-red colour. Convolutions dark gray, with an evident tinge of dull red. On squeezing convolutions, livid-red puncta became very evident and numerous. Medullary substance studded with large dark puncta; linear coagula few. Corpus callosum and fornix healthy, the latter remarkably small. Both thalami small, of a darker colour than usual; both have large puncta and broad blood-channels in their interior. The right thalamus is a fourth larger than the left. Neither thalamus is appreciably softened. Hygrometric vesicles in choroid plexuses. Commissura mollis intact, healthy. Right corpus striatum rather larger than left; both healthy. Corpora albicantia small, but healthy. Pituitary body, infundibulum and tuber cinereum normal. Pons varolii,

sedative alkaloids of opium, and, being an aqueous solution, is quite free from narcotine. A genial and certain sedative, it very seldom produces constipation or headache and, more rarely than any other opiate, vomiting.

in its interior, of a remarkably dark colour, and full of livid puncta; neither it nor the medulla oblongata softened. Arteries collapsed, opposed surfaces in contact. No blood in basilar, vertebral, or cerebral arteries. The right pupil was, as in life, markedly contracted.

CASE VII.—E. T—, æt. 46, single, a domestic servant; admitted March 5th, 1855, from Brighton.

A sallow, dusky-complexioned woman, of average height and slight frame; extremely emaciated and feeble. Skin cool. Facial expression good, but fatuous and unvarying. Pupils unequal, right the larger, both very sluggish. Nostrils markedly compressed, not unequal. Upper lip long and straight. Tongue large, flabby, and tremulous. Gait feeble and devious. Utterance very defective and slow. Hands cold and livid. Pulse 104, very feeble.

Her memory is annihilated. She is entirely ignorant of and indifferent to her present deplorable condition. She is depressed, but free from delusion.

Stated to have been insane six months; her insanity is attributed to "disappointment in marriage."

There is a slough on the left natis.

Her mental symptoms did not vary from those above described, except that she had occasionally melancholic delusions; thus, she once said, "My sisters would go crazy if they knew I was going to be killed;" and sometimes she imagined she was poisoned, and sometimes starved. This latter delusion she had while her lips were yet wet with porter, with which, and with other nourishing food, she was liberally supplied. The nocturnal accessions of paralytic mania were very evident. The right pupil continued the larger till her death, which happened on March 21st, 1855. After a restless night she became comatose and motionless at 1 a.m.; never rallying, she died at 9 a.m.

Autopsy, seventy-eight hours after death.—Body extremely emaciated. Scalp peeled off easily, bloodless. Skull thin. Brain small. Dura mater and arachnoid healthy. Subarachnoid and inter-convolutional serum copious. Pia mater congested. Convolutional neurine thin and bloodless.

Medullary substance of hemispheres studded with numerous large, livid puncta. Ventricles full of serum. Corpus callosum decidedly soft to the stream; fornix softer than the corpus callosum. Corpora striata and optic thalami very small, else normal. Crura cerebri, at their junction with the pons, broken off in getting the brain out, though no force was used in so doing. The interior of the crura was diffluent. Arteries are full of dark blood, their coats thicker and more rigid than normal; their cut orifices are not widely patent.

CASE VIII.—J. H—, æt. 65, married, a fisherman ; admitted June 5th, 1855.

A tall, deaf man, of strong frame, emaciated, and in an extremely feeble physical condition. Skin hottish. Facial expression apprehensive, fatuous, and with the peculiar listening look of the deaf. Eyes gray ; pupils contracted, nearly insensible, very irregular. Pulse 84, full, from marked arterial rigidity. Tongue large, and slightly tremulous ; utterance not affected. His gait is very feeble, and his progression difficult from old injury of the hip. He is utterly incoherent, abusive and obscene in language, but not violent or depressed. He is stated to have been insane two months. Cause unknown. Ext. Hyoscy. ℈j, h. s,

June 11th.—Till to-day he has been noisy, abusive, and obscene. He is now depressed and hypochondriacal, snivelling or vociferating at fancied pain ; " prays the Almighty to take his life." From June 11th till within a few days of his death he was alternately apprehensive, morose, and disgustingly abusive ; or well-disposed, amiable, and polite. While in the former condition his language was quite a curiosity of Billingsgate ; in the latter, he repeated his prayers aloud, sang hymns, was grateful for everything done for him, and made himself, as far as lay in his power, agreeable. The former condition, however, predominated. Died of exhaustion, November 27th, 1855, after three days' semi-coma.

Autopsy, five hours after death.—Scalp bloodless ; skull of normal thickness. Middle meningeal artery full of dark-coloured blood; dura mater strongly adherent to vault. Half an inch to the right of the confluence of the coronal and sagittal sutures, and in the frontal bone, was a deep diaphanous depression, large enough to contain a horse-bean. Arachnoid adherent along the mesian longitudinal line of the hemispheres, here and there slightly opaque; sub-arachnoid fluid copious; the quantity of fluid in the *cavity* of the arachnoid marked; pia mater peels off easily. Arteries quite free from atheroma, full of dark-coloured blood; convolutions thin, dark, not congested. Puncta large, numerous, and dark, more conspicuous in right than in left centrum ovale. Linear coagula in the vessels of right hemisphere numerous. Ventricles full of serum. Corpus callosum normal; the fornix descending from its raphé very thin, tough, and semitransparent; it resembles thin bladder, and can be pulled out, without injury, to the width of an inch. It is not white, but of a dirty grayish hue. The fornix, lower surface of corpus callosum, corpora striata, and optic thalami, covered with minute, transparent vesicles, like sudamina; they do not feel rough or gritty to the finger, but their elevation is very perceptible. Optic thalami small, equal, of normal consistence. The puncta of the right are numerous and dark. The gray matter of both extremely dark. Corpora striata normal, equal. Commissura mollis very firm, and of a dark pinkish-gray colour. Corpora albicantia small, pure white and firm; medulla oblongata remarkably small. No softening anywhere.

CASE IX.—J. B—, æt. 30, single, a cabinet-maker; admitted November 7th, 1855, from London.

A pale, sallow man, of middle height and average frame, rather emaciated, in a feeble physical condition. Skin cool; expression fatuous, unvarying, neither elated nor depressed. Eyes hazel; pupils contracted, unequal, left slightly the more contracted. Nostrils normal. Tongue large, livid, very tremulous; utterance nearly unintelligible. Gait rather feeble. Upper lip long, straight, unchiselled. Pulse extremely feeble.

He is highly excited and elated; walks jauntily or runs;

demented and incoherent. From his imperfect articulation, it is difficult to make out what his exact delusions are. He is reported to be dangerous.

History none, except that he has been insane three weeks.

Ext. Hyoscy. gr. xv, h. s.

November 8th.—Ext. Hyoscy. Əj, h. s.

9th.—All his elation has disappeared ; he is now somewhat depressed.

10th.—Depressed.

11th.—Tranquil.

13th.—Has been highly destructive in the night, tearing his sheets and night-dress. Continue Ext. Hyoscy. Əj, bis die.

14th.—Tranquil and orderly, walking in airing ground.

From this date to the day of his death, February 1st, 1856, he was nearly constantly the subject of horrible and extravagant delusions. When in bed (as he often was), he usually pulled the clothes over his head to protect himself from " the bloody thieves and murderers " who, he fancied, in thousands surrounded him, and sometimes to ward off their blows and the " twenty-thousand books they were throwing at him." He often refused his food from delusion of poisoning, and was frequently snivelling and whining, he could not say why. Sometimes he imagined he was " full of horses' bones," and that a " great surgeon from the skies " had already taken four pounds of bones out of his chest. This frightful state of depression was on three or four occasions relieved by gleams of elated fancy. He then said he had " a great diamond in his head," and iterated sonorously and for hours " hundreds and thousands and millions." The pupils, which were usually dilated by extract of henbane, of which he frequently took half a drachm twice and sometimes thrice a day, were nearly constantly unequal, the right being markedly the larger. During his gleams of elation they were equal or nearly so. At noon on January 31st, having been gradually reduced to mere skin and bone by the intensity of his excitement, he became motionless and insensible. At 8 a.m. on February 1st he expired. During the

and fourteen hours of life his breathing was so feeble and
interrupted, that it was sometimes difficult to say whether
he was alive or dead, a state of uncertainty only cleared up
by an occasional feeble respiration.

Autopsy, six hours after death.—Scalp bloodless, tough ;
skull of natural thickness and consistence. Dura mater
normal, except concave edge of falx, which is anteriorly
thin and reticular. Arachnoid normal; there are a few
old slight adhesions along the sagittal margin of hemispheres ; sub-arachnoid serum trifling. Through the arachnoid the surface of the right hemisphere looked of a buff-gray,
and was certainly much lighter in colour than the surface of
the left. The right convolutions were fewer and shallower
than the left, and pia mater did not strip off easily. Puncta
in the left centrum ovale normal in number, but largish and
livid; in the right centrum ovale morbidly few and pale.
Cortical substance of right hemisphere pale and bloodless.
Little or no serum in ventricles ; corpus callosum normal.
Vertical part of fornix thin and diaphanous ; horizontal part
narrow ; halves equal, not soft. Right thalamus and corpus
striatum decidedly smaller than the left. Blood-vessels on
these bodies few, pale and small, those on the corresponding
left structures being normally numerous, bright, and large.
Section of the thalami and corpora striata proved that the
right ganglia were at least a fourth the smaller ; the inner
structure of the right thalamus was nearly bloodless, the
left had the usual number of exuding livid puncta ; neither
thalami nor corpora striata were softened or altered in consistence. Commissura mollis small, soft, and would evidently
have soon broken down. Corpora albicantia equal, normal,
but small ; not softened. Arteries collapsed, quite free
from atheroma, contained some dark fluid blood. Vesicular
substance of pons varolii slate-gray, bloodless, hard. Medulla oblongata hardish, bloodless. Cerebellum healthy,
softer (as usual) than the cerebrum.

Case X.—W. F—, æt. 35, widower, a labourer from
Sussex ; admitted July 25th, 1855.

A fair, fatuous-looking man, of average height and strong

frame, rather emaciated, in a feeble physical condition. Skin cool. Facial expression neither elated nor depressed, unvarying. Eyes gray. Pupils contracted, feebly sensitive; right pupil slightly irregular. Nostrils unequal; the right the smaller. Mouth broad; upper lip long, straight, and nearly devoid of curves. Tongue large, livid, tremulous, furred white. Bowels confined; abdomen not tense. Pulse 76, full, from slight arterial rigidity. Gait feeble.

He is good tempered and cheerful, but incoherent and demented. Has no delusion. The duration of the attack (the first) is stated to be "one month." Its cause, "drinking and natural imbecility." From the day of his admission to that of his death the type of his mental symptoms varied, at short intervals, from snivelling depression and apprehensiveness to childish elation. When elated, he talked in the peculiar endearing tone which mothers and nurses often employ in talking to children. His habits were destructive, though not very so, and his incoherent dementia complete. During the last four months of life he nearly constantly ground his teeth. The pupils, except when dilated by Hyoscyamus, were equal, contracted, and slightly irregular. Getting rapidly feebler and more emaciated, at 7 p.m. on the 14th of February, 1856, he became comatose and motionless. At 10 p.m. the face twitched, and the otherwise motionless coma was profound. At 2½ a.m. on the 15th of February he expired.

Autopsy, twelve hours after death.—Body very emaciated. Scalp bloodless, peeled off easily. Skull thin, dense. Temporal muscles large and fleshy. Calvarium capacious, the brain did not appear to fill it, especially anteriorly. Dura mater attached with unusual firmness to vault. Falx cerebri reticular anteriorly. Arachnoid slightly adherent at the sagittal border of hemispheres. Cortex, seen through arachnoid, unhealthily white. Vessels of pia mater few, pale, and flaccid. Sub-arachnoid serum trifling. Pia mater palish, stripped off easily. Cortex thin, buff-gray, with a conspicuous white line, parallel to and following the windings of the convolutions, in its centre. Convolutions remarkably shallow. The white part of the centra ovalia very large. Puncta normal, livid. Ventricles distended by serum. Corpus callosum and fornix softish. Halves of fornix equal. The commissure itself well developed, its posterior extremity being two inches wide. Velum inter-positum and plexus choroides normal, but unusually pale. Thalami optici and corpora striata rather small, but equal, and of normal consistence. The third ventricle normally closed. Commissura mollis thin. The blood-vessels on right side of septum lucidum, on the right corpus striatum, in the right descending cornu, much paler, and many fewer than on the corresponding left structures. Interior of the right thalamus and corpus striatum pale, bloodless, and grooved, with many empty channels. Interior of left thalamus and left corpus striatum with the normal number of livid puncta. Fourth ventricle and optic tubercles healthy. Pons varolii and medulla oblongata normally hard. Cerebellum normally soft. Arteries at base free from atheroma, but full of dark clots. Corpora albicantia small, but otherwise normal. Crura cerebri, tuber cinereum, infundibulum, and pituitary body, healthy. Pupils mark-edly contracted. Rigor mortis slight. Brachial artery full of liquid blood, cut ends quite patent, its caliber undi-minished.

CASE XI.—E. B—, æt. 37, a gamekeeper's wife, from near Chichester; admitted September 21st, 1855.

A florid, emaciated woman, above the middle height, of average frame, in feeble physical condition. Skin cool; hands clammy. Cheeks livid red; small vessels separately injected. Facial expression extremely depressed. Eyes brown; pupils very contracted, irregular, and feebly sensi-tive; right pupil the more irregular, its axis diverging. Nostrils equal, alæ markedly contracted at their superior edge. Upper lip long, straight, not quite destitute of chiselling. Mouth broad; lips livid. Tongue rather tre-mulous, flabby, and livid. Gait very feeble. Utterance not affected. Pulse 88, feeble, but sharpish. Bowels, she says, not open, and that she is sleepless and has strong epigastric pulsation, which, however, cannot be felt.

She is not incoherent, but extremely depressed, and the subject of melancholic delusions; imagines she is about to die, and is convinced that she "will not get better;" says that a week since she "threatened to strangle herself, as she thought she should never die, and that, when she attempts to pray, all manner of deranged people appear to her and say, ' You shan't die.' "

She attributes her condition to the deaths of her brother-in-law and niece five months ago. Her aunt died insane.

She was in tolerable health until she went to attend on her brother-in-law during his illness. The hysterical demonstrations of his widow were noticed to have an extraordinarily depressing effect on her. On returning home from her brother-in-law's funeral, the first patently insane idea was noticed. She suddenly fancied she had a sore on her tongue, and insisted on her husband examining it; and though constantly told there was no sore, she as constantly reasserted its existence. During the five months from the funeral to the day of admission, she has steadily become more depressed. Liq. Opii, ♏xl, o. n.

22d.—Slept fairly and looks much better this morning.

23d.—Eyeballs yellow. Pil. Col. c. Cal., and Liq. Opii, ♏l, h. s.

25th.—Scleroticæ still tinged. Has erratic hypochondriacal pains (particularly in hip and ankle) and hysterical sensations. Bowels confined. Tongue large, livid, and tremulous. Pupils continue contracted and irregular. Haust. Sennæ, f ℥iss, c. Pil. Col. c. Cal. Continue Liq. Opii, ♏l, o. n.

26th.—Bowels open. Fancies she can't swallow, and takes nauseous physic only by sips. Rep. haust. Sennæ, f ℥ij, c. Cal. c. Opio.

27th.—Bowels well relieved; swallows better to-day.

28th.—Says her " heart beats so, that she is obliged to

hold her ribs lest it should beat through." There is no abnormal cardiac pulsation. Continue Liq. Opii, ♏l, o. n.

October 1st.—Hypochondriacal sensations continue. Eyeballs still yellow. Emp. Belladonnæ regioni cordis; Pil. Col. c. Cal. j, statim.

3d.—Pil. Hyd. c. Col. j, alternis noctibus.

4th.—Says there is "something wrong with her water, and that she sometimes does not pass any for weeks." Liq. Opii, ʒj, o. n.

12th.—She is more cheerful and industrious at needle-work. Eyeballs less yellow; pupils as heretofore. Continue Pil. alternis noctibus, and Liq. Opii, ʒj, o. n.

November 14th.—Has been since last note very depressed, and full of imaginary ailments and sensations. She is markedly worse; fancies a "spirit comes to her bedside and scratches;" it says, "Your husband is married again; you shall never sleep." "You shall live till you are skin and bone," &c. Omit Pill; continue Liq. Opii, ʒj, o. n.

December 21st.—Since last note she has gradually become worse. She is now to the last degree depressed, full of horrible delusions, and only takes food on being fed. On the 26th of November, for two hours in the afternoon, she had an extraordinary burst of hilarity; she was, during that time, elated, singing, dancing, talking to and mimicking all the people in the room. She afterwards became very low. As a reason for her previous mirth, said she "heard a voice saying, ' Be merry before you go.' " She is now extremely emaciated and feeble. The pupils are contracted, irregular, and nearly fixed. Continue Liq. Opii, ʒj, o. n.

January 3d, 1856.—Intense melancholia continues; she has become, however, very taciturn, so that her delusions are not very apparent. Gets daily more attenuated and feeble; takes food only on being persuasively fed. Discontinue Liq. Opii.

March 4th.—Since last note has been, in consequence of her increasing feebleness, in bed. During the interval has been constantly frightfully depressed, and often the subject of horrible delusions; imagines she "has committed murder and adultery," that her "bones will never be buried," &c. She is often restless, getting in or out of bed, and attempting to run down stairs, in the hope, apparently, of escaping. She is a living skeleton from emaciation; unless food be forced on her, she will not take it, yet at times, for an hour or two, she will demand food and eat ravenously. It appears physically impossible that she can hold together for many more days, or even hours.

18th.—Remained in the same condition till 7 p.m. to-day, when she became motionless and insensible. Corneæ glazed; pupils contracted.

19th.—Died at 4.45 a.m.

Autopsy, ten hours after death.—Scalp perfectly bloodless, easily torn down. Skull thin, extremely brittle. Two pits observed on interior of calvarium, of unequal size, similarly placed in either half of the skull, namely, at the anterior mesian angle of each parietal bone, a quarter of an inch from the confluence of the coronal and sagittal sutures; the channel of the arteria meningea media ran into each pit; this was particularly evident on the left side, where, also, the pit was larger, being of the dimensions of a large horse-bean. The pit on the right side, divided by a ridge of bone, would more properly be described as two adjacent pits, each large enough to contain a small split pea. The whole skull was more or less diaphanous, but at the pits it was quite transparent. Dura mater and arachnoid healthy. The ordinary paccionian adhesion of the arachnoid surfaces existed along the posterior sagittal edge of the hemispheres. Sub-arachnoid serum copious. Many ounces of serum, escaping through a rent in the base of the third ventricle (tuber cinereum), flowed into the cavity of the arachnoid. Structures at base all softish, some diffluent. Corpora albicantia soft, but retaining their contour, though not quite their colour. Right corpus albicans the smaller. In tracing the right optic nerve over its corresponding crus cerebri, the inferior aspect of the middle lobe was found to be diffluent, and the descending cornu of the right lateral ventricle was thus unintentionally laid open. No similar condition observable on the left side. Arteries of the base normal, free from atheroma, collapsed, and not distended by blood. Pia mater peeled off convolutions easily. Cortex normal, bloodless. Centra ovalia have few puncta. Corpus callosum normal superiorly. On laying open the lateral ventricles, the most curious appearance I have ever seen in the diseased brain presented itself. The fornix, no longer attached to the lower raphé of the corpus callosum, lay, or rather what remained of it lay, a shapeless, diffluent mass, deep between the thalami, in fact, in the third ventricle. Velum interpositum there was none, nor any trace of the commissura mollis. The difference in the size and the planes of the thalami and corpora striata was most remarkable, the left thalamus being, at least, twice as large as, and half an inch higher than, the right. This difference, though very obvious between the corpora striata, was not so marked as between the thalami. The upper part of either thalamus was little altered in consistence, but their bases, which form the lower part of the cleft and the floor of the third ventricle, were markedly though unequally changed. The whole base of the right thalamus was diffluent, that of the left softish, but not in a condition approaching diffluence. The disintegration of the base of the right thalamus explains the difference of the thalamic planes. The anterior commissure was very oblique, and the right pillar of the fornix entered the base of its thalamus nearly half an inch lower than the corresponding left pillar. Neither corpus striatum was altered in consistence. The anterior wall of the right descending ventricular cornu was diffluent; the posterior wall, including the pes hippocampi, hippocampus major, &c., was normal. Left descending cornu softish, but otherwise normal. Right crus cerebri soft; fourth ventricle softish. Pons varolii the hardest part of the encephalon. Cerebellum and medulla oblongata normal.

CASE XII.—Female, name unknown, æt. about 40; history unknown. Some days ago she was brought by the

police to the City of London Union-house, as a wandering
lunatic; admitted April 14th, 1856.

A sallow woman, of middle height, average frame, tolerably
well nourished, and in fair physical condition. Skin cool.
Facial expression cunning, semifatuous, and merry. Eyes
brown; pupils unequal, contracted, very feebly sensitive;
left pupil rather the larger, right the more irregular. Nostrils equal, large, shapeless. Tongue normal, clean. Pulse
100, sharpish, but easily put out by the finger. Gait
normal. The wrists, forearms, and legs are discoloured by
bruises, the result of recent mechanical restraint. She has
lost, or feigns to have lost, the power of intelligible articulation; nevertheless she pronounces some words perfectly,
such as "Yes, sir," at the commencement of an answer;
but then, as if recollecting she was betraying herself, commences talking volubly an utterly unintelligible childish gibberish. When asked to come up stairs to have her case
taken, said distinctly, "I'll have my tea first." Various
plans were tried to induce her to speak intelligibly, and
to extract from her her name; to no purpose however.
She remained in the same condition till the 2d of May.
During the interval she often articulated distinctly oaths
and short sentences. Thus, on coming from the bath, she
alluded and pointed to her discoloured arms and legs;
and, on one occasion, being taken round the female depart-
ment by Mr. Austin, said to the attendant, "I have been
for a walk with the doctor." She was usually restless,
cheerfully talking her gibberish, and laughing fatuously.
More rarely she was spiteful and violent, and occasionally
dirty in her habits. At 7 a.m. on the 2d of May, having
been quiet all night, she was discovered to be comatose and
motionless. Anæsthesia, as regards the fingers, arms, and
hands, complete. Soles insensible to tickling, but the
movements of the legs are lively on pinching the toes.
Eyelids closed, pupils markedly contracted; no stertor or
puffing of lips. Enema salis, statim. She has had three
epileptiform seizures up to noon. The left upper eyelid,
left side of face, left arm and leg, were strongly convulsed,
the corresponding parts on the right side remaining quite

passive. In the interval between the fits either arm falls a
dead weight. Left pupil markedly dilated, right pupil as
markedly contracted; both are insensible. The condition
of tactual sensation the same as described as existing at
7 a.m. Bowels open freely both before and after the saline
enema. Motions not lumpy. Continue the salt injection.
—5 p.m. Fits continue at intervals of a few minutes. No
scream, but marked teeth-grinding. The first symptom of
the seizure is the sudden turning up of the eyeballs obliquely towards the left. Both arms and both legs are
now convulsed, but the left arm and leg conspicuously the
more so. During the interval anæsthesia is everywhere
profound. Continue enema salis.—9 p.m. Fits continue.
Anæsthesia and paralysis universal. Mucous rattle in
bronchi loud. She is apparently moribund.

May 3d, 9 a.m.—Has been in fits more or less all night.
Right eyelids glued together; left eyelids open and free
from adhesive secretion; the eyeballs feebly roll; right
pupil markedly contracted, left as markedly dilated. Coma
is much less profound, and the facial expression much less
vacant. Paralysis everywhere complete. Anæsthesia has
disappeared. Tickling of the soles produces slight, pinching
of the toes lively, movements. Continue enemata.—2½ p.m.
Fits continue. In articulo mortis. Died at 3.15 p.m.

Autopsy, twenty hours after death.—Rigor mortis normal,
less in the upper than in the lower extremities. Both
pupils dilated, left the larger. Scalp peeled off readily;
livid posteriorly with liquid flood. Skull immensely thick
anteriorly; quite opaque everywhere except at the sutures
and the paccionian depressions; frontal bones half an inch
thick anteriorly, and very dense in texture; anterior
cranial cavity contracted, shelving, and generally disproportionably small; dura mater not adherent to calvarium.
Arachnoid healthy; the usual paccionian adhesions exist.
Pia mater, which strips readily off convolutions, is rather
livid and congested. Surface-veins not abnormally numerous or distended, but very dark coloured. Subarachnoid and interconvolutional serum most marked, and
evidently stretching and raising the arachnoid. Brain very

small, especially so anteriorly. Convolutions are fewer, less sinuous and deep than usual. Puncta of centra ovalia few and livid. Corpus callosum, fornix, and velum interpositum normal. Commissura mollis thin and soft, nearly diffluent. Left thalamus and corpus striatum rather smaller than the right, which are apparently healthy. The anterior thalamic eminence does not exist on the left side, though marked on the right. Left thalamus and corpus striatum are softer, their internal structure much less distinct, and the gray matter of a much lighter colour than in the corresponding ganglia on the right side. In the substance of the left thalamus are numerous empty blood-channels, and many vessels blocked up with long, thread-like, whitish clots of fibrin, the absence of exuding puncta and the general bloodlessness of the ganglion being at the same time remarkable. The right thalamus and corpus striatum healthy in consistence, in distinctness of striæ, and supply of blood.

Basic structures normal, with the exception of the corpora albicantia, which are of a dirty buff colour, soft nearly to diffluence; their outline very indistinct. The left is the smaller, the less regular in contour, and the more nearly diffluent. The sides of the fissura sylvii are incompletely agglutinated, so that in tracing the middle cerebral artery the gray matter is ruptured and torn off with the pia mater. Both internal carotids markedly patent and atheromatous. Vertebrals patent, their coats thicker than normal, but not atheromatous. At the bifurcation of the basilar into the posterior cerebrals there is a large distinct patch of atheroma. All the arterial tubes are to the finger thicker and harder, and to the eye more opaque than usual. The cavity of the arachnoid at base full of serum, from the rupture of the floor of the third ventricle. Infundibulum, pituitary body, and tuber cinereum quite healthy. Pons varolii and medulla oblongata are, as normally, the hardest, and the cerebellum the softest healthy part of the encephalon. Spinal marrow healthily hard, as far as it could be traced from the skull. From the spinal canal flowed a copious serum on the dependance of the head. The petrous portion of the right temporal bone was brittle, cancellous, and much softer than the left;

the right tympanic cavity being laid open by the end of the ordinary forceps, impelled by the least tap of a mallet. The right ossicula auditus were thus extracted intact. No similar softening or brittleness on left side. The right superior semicircular canal could not be laid open by the knife. No appearance of necrosed bone in either temporal region.

Case XIII.—J. J—, a surgeon, æt. 40, a private patient, unmarried; admitted September, 1854.

A tall fair man of average frame, emaciated, in feeble health. Skin cool; complexion highly coloured, the tint a dusky red. Tongue tremulous, flabby, red, and clean. Bowels are open. Pulse feeble, unequal in beat and in power. Arteries slightly rigid. Expression of face un-varying, fatuous, neither indicative of good or bad spirits; face destitute of lines. Lips tremulous, especially the upper lip. Nostrils unequal, right markedly the larger, tremulous and shapeless. Eyes gray, arcus senilis conspicuous; right pupil markedly contracted and insensible; left round, dilated, and extremely sluggish. Gait tottery and devious. Utterance halting, but very distinct.

He is partially incoherent, very inconsecutive, and rather elated. The memory is greatly impaired. He jumbles in following sentences, ideas and facts connected with totally different subjects. His only marked delusions are, that Shakspeare and Milton died respectively at the ages of 156 and 112.

His attack is stated to be of nine months' date. There is no doubt, however, that it has been coming on for at least eighteen months, as a year and a half ago he suddenly commenced singing vociferously at church, and was guilty of numerous extravagances, which were totally foreign to his usual tranquil and unobtrusive demeanour. Three years ago he was severely injured about the head in a railway accident. He is stated to have received a blow on the left side of the head, to have had bleeding from the left ear, and to have been insensible for an hour after the injury. When seen by the surgeon of the company, a few days after the accident, he had partial deafness of the left ear, partial paralysis of the left facial muscles, and inability to close the left eyelids. The mouth was drawn to the right. All these symptoms disappeared shortly afterwards. His history is one of disappointed hopes in his profession, of frequent changes, and as many failures.

27th.—Busily employed in writing out passages from the "Epistles."

October 7th.—Has no idea where he is : says Mr. B——, a demented patient, "should be removed to a lunatic asylum." Since his admission has abstained from, and cannot be induced to take meat, from his conviction of the truth of "Vegetarianism." He continues somewhat elated.

13th.—Large delusions are more evident ; talks of some gentleman's seven wives, and of this person's intention to marry another lady.

20th.—His notions enlarge. Says he is "going to Australia in the 'Leviathan' ship building by Mr. Scott Russell," and that during the "first month after his arrival in the colonies he shall send £100,000 to his father." He has abandoned vegetarianism.

January 13th, 1855.—Continues elated. He is now full of all manner of absurd schemes. Left pupil remains widely dilated, and the right markedly contracted. Both are insensible. The physical condition has greatly improved.

February 16th.—Has become more noisy and excited ; he is consequently feebler and more emaciated. His schemes and ideas are all of a large type.

April 2d.—He gets feebler. His large delusions alternate with melancholic ones. Says the Earl and Countess of D—— are dead, &c. The left pupil at these periods is much less dilated than usual.

May 31st.—Continues to get feebler. The delusions are scarcely noticeable. Left pupil always, though not uniformly, the larger.

October 22d.—Is much improved physically, and has been so during the last three months. Goes out in Victoria Park frequently for a couple of hours' walk. Irritable, somewhat elated, and partially incoherent. He has no apparent delusion. The right pupil is fixed and contracted, the left the larger, and feebly sensitive.

March 1st, 1856.—He is not more lost or feeble, nor has he been since last note. Has no large delusion. He is irritable and interfering, but not badly disposed. Pupils remain as heretofore.

4th.—Yesterday at 3·45 p.m. became suddenly stupid and speechless. In a minute or two, though still speechless, he became restless and perverse. He now insisted on buttoning all his fellow patients' coats, and arranging their neckties. Ol. Ricini, ʒj, statim.

5th.—Bowels well open: is now incoherently talkative concerning his relations. No change in the condition of the pupils.

6th.—Continues very stupid and irritable. Ol. Croton, ℳj, statim.—8 p.m. Bowels freely relieved.

7th.—Less stupid, but very feeble and tottery.

19th.—Is at times extremely heavy and stupid.

20th.—Bewildered and ill-tempered, persists in undressing himself.

26th.—Has grand delusions to-day: talking of the " 400,000,000 sovereigns he possesses."

April 18th.—Is sometimes volubly talkative of his supposed riches, and at other times obstinately silent. The pupils are as heretofore.

April 26th, 1856.—When seen at 0·45 p.m. would not speak, though pressed to do so. At 1 p.m. he dined; walked to the dinner-table, helped himself to roast beef, of which he ate heartily; then took some rice pudding. He had nearly finished his plateful, when he suddenly fell back insensible in his chair, and being taken into an adjoining room died in three or four minutes from the moment of seizure. The pupils were equally and widely dilated during the last minute of life.

Autopsy, seventy-two hours after death.—Body in good condition, legs and abdomen fleshy. Rigor mortis slight in upper, and less than usual in lower extremities. Marked stasis on posterior aspect of body. Ears very livid, but can be squeezed white. Pupils not equal, right rather the smaller; both dilated. Scalp very thick and dense, gorged with dark blood, and difficult to detach. Skull thick, dense, not brittle. The inner cranial surface presented a very singular appearance; its temporal, parietal, and frontal regions were marked with a minute and peculiar red tracery of bone; here and there it presented a warty appearance, like the surface of the verucous growths of the penis. The whole cranial surface was similarly but less evidently marked, and was conspicuous for its high glaze, so that the polished tracery looked in many places like tesselated pavement on a small scale. Skull immensely thick, and everywhere opaque. The petrous portion of neither temporal bone deserved its name, it being composed of large and brittle cancelli, which in both bones were, from their extreme thinness, quite transparent; the right temporal surface was the more so, and the internal cancellous structure was distinctly seen through it. The least touch of the knife laid open the cavity of the tympanum, and one cut of a blunt scalpel was sufficient to lay bare in its whole length the cavity of the superior semicircular canal. The other canals preserved something of their normal hardness. The cancellous degeneration was generally less evident on the left side: though the left tympanic cavity was laid open by one touch of the knife, neither the semicircular canals, nor any other part of the left acoustic apparatus, was very evidently altered in consistence. The ossicula auditus were on both sides healthy. The left side of calvarium, and the left cerebellar impression, were certainly the larger; and just to the right of the confluence of occipital channels was a deep conoidal pit, of the size of a small bean; the cranium was not transparent at this spot. The dura mater, thick, fibrous, and very glistening, was scarcely at all attached to the vault, though normally so to the base of the skull. Arachnoid healthy; the usual trifling paccionian adhesions alone existing. The surface of the brain was but little livid with turgid veins. Subarachnoid serum very marked. Pia mater, which stripped clean off the cortex, was minutely injected and very livid. The brain, which evidently did not fill the skull, was small, and its convolutions fewer and shallower than natural. Gray cortical substance softish and rather injected. Centra ovalia marked with numerous livid, non-exuding puncta. All the medullary vessels were filled with large linear, livid clots; every part of the brain presented this appearance. Corpus callosum normal. On raising the great commissure, the whole body of the fornix, being quite diffluent, separated from it. The anterior pillars of the fornix were very soft, and did not retain their rounded outline. Septum lucidum and hippocampi, &c., healthy. The body of the fornix could not be raised from the velum interpositum, but had to be scraped off that membrane, which was intact and normal. Commissura mollis none, nor any vestige of it. Right thalamus at least one third smaller than left. No change of consistence in either, but both were studded with numerous clot-puncta. The sides of the fissura Sylvii were glued together, so that there was some difficulty in tracing the middle cerebral arteries. The bases of both middle lobes, forming the floors of the descending ventricular cornua, were equally soft, but not in a condition approaching diffluence. A very little and tender manipulation sufficed to expose each pes hippocampi. Arteries of base normal and full of livid blood. Pons healthily hard. The lower extremity of pons separated from medulla oblongata, which was decidedly soft, in getting out the brain. Cerebellum, as usual, the softest part of the healthy encephalon. A copious serum escaped from a rupture of the floor of the third ventricle.

CASE XIV.—R. V—, æt. 46, married, a porter, and in the habit of carrying heavy weights on his head; admitted January 28th, 1856.

A short man, of strongish frame, in feeble physical condition, though tolerably well nourished. Complexion fair, naturally coloured. Facial expression neither that of elation or dejection; no play of feature. Eyes gray; pupils round, equal, sensitive. Nostrils equal. Tongue large, flabby, hard, not tremulous. Utterance of consonants imperfect. Mouth broad; upper lip long, straight, nearly devoid of chiselling. Pulse 96, sharpish. Gait straddling and rather feeble. He is utterly incoherent, intensely excited, elated, restless, and full of the grandest delusions of wealth and rank.

The cause of his malady is unknown. His wife ascribes it to his getting wet through in December, 1854, and remaining, while exhausted by fatigue, in his dripping clothes. During the last year his manner has completely altered; from being gentle and considerate, he has become irritable, selfish, and even morose. During the last four months he has been evidently insane; the first three months he was at home, full of grand delusions of wealth, and constantly talking of the immense sum he was collecting for the queen to carry on the war with. During the last month he has been in the workhouse, where his habits have become destructive, and himself savage and violent. When admitted he had two frightful black eyes. Ext. Hyoscy. Əj, h. s.

29th.—Ext. Hyoscy. ʒss, o. n. Takes food well. Continues highly excited.

30th.—Full of the largest fancies, restless, and making the oddest gestures and grimaces. Ext. Hyoscy. ʒss, bis die.

February 1st.—Is much more tranquil.

3d.—And continues so.

5th.—Tranquil. Continue Ext. Hyoscy. ʒss, bis die. Pupils dilated wide.

12th.—Continues to be calmed by the henbane.

From 13th to 18th.—Had diarrhœa, which was checked by the Pil. Cupri c. Opio (Cupri Sulph. Pulv. Opii āā gr. ss), 6tis horis. Between these dates the henbane was omitted; as a consequence he became intensely excited.

19th.—Ext. Hyoscy. ʒss, semel die.

20th.—Ext. Hyoscy. ʒss, bis die.

23d.—Much quieter, gently under the influence of henbane.

26th.—The excitement becoming more intense, the Extract was given in Əij doses twice a day. From this date to the 19th of June, he continued to be daily maniacally excited; the character of his delusions being as often horrible as pleasant. Of whatever type the fancies were, they were always highly coloured. During the prevalence of melancholic delusions, he was morose and horribly abusive, violent in gesture, and destructive in habit. When his fancies were pleasurable, he was good-tempered, laughed, sang, and danced with maniacal energy. In either condition the excitement nearly daily rose to the highest pitch. The only means of calming him was the administration of two scruples of the Ext. Hyoscyami. This dose he usually took twice, often thrice, a day. The pupils were always and equally dilated. From the intense excitement he gradually became feeble and emaciated, though his appetite was good and he was well sustained by a liberal diet.

On the 8th of June, the intense excitement continuing, he was kept in bed, in consequence of his advancing feebleness. He remained in bed till the 19th of June. At 1 p.m. on that day he was snorting, like a steam-engine blowing off its steam, and at half-past one he was singing maniacally. At 2 p.m. he became tranquil. From this time he was never seen to move voluntarily, or heard to speak. At 9 p.m. he was lying on the left side, in a condition of profound coma, of universal anæsthesia and paralysis. The eyelids were half-open, and the eyeballs feebly rolled. The pupils markedly and equally contracted and insensible. The feet powerfully inverted and crossed. The arms were crossed on the chest, and the wrists curiously distorted; the hands being pronated to their utmost extent, and forcibly everted. The forearms, if uncrossed, by degrees convulsively re-crossed each other on the chest. Abdominal respiration was nearly annihilated, and the retraction of the abdominal wall most marked, thoracic respiration being sufficiently evident. There was no movement of the sterno-cleido-mastoidei. He was very wet and dirty from urine and fæces. Died at midnight.

Autopsy, twenty hours after death.—Body very emaciated. Pupils markedly dilated. Rigor mortis slight, scarcely any in the arms. Scalp thin, nearly bloodless, easily torn down. Skull of normal consistence, thin, and everywhere diaphanous, especially so at the paccionian pits in the right parietal bone. Inner surface of calvarium not conspicuously marked with arterial impressions; skull easily separable from dura mater, which was quite healthy. Arachnoid normal; the usual paccionian adhesions existed. Pia mater congested, brightish red, did not peel clean off cortex. Convolutions of a healthy colour and consistence, but somewhat shallow, and hardly as sinuous as usual. Centra ovalia of unequal size, the left being manifestly the larger. Puncta below the average in number, bright-red, and non-exuding. All the medullary substance studded with numerous linear, red, fibrin-clots. In the act of removing the brain, a jet of yellow-ish serum issued from the outer and lower part of the right hemisphere, just about the junction of the middle and posterior lobes. Corpus callosum normal in appearance and size, but softer than usual. On raising the great transverse commissure, the whole fornix was found to be diffluent, and lying as a semi-fluid amorphous layer on the velum interpositum; the septum lucidum was disintegrated, and no longer recognisable. The only parts of the fornix not completely broken down were its anterior pillars and the cornua ammonis; of the pillars, both of which were very soft, the left was the softer, and on a lower plane than the right. The anterior commissure was soft, on the verge of diffluence, and oblique, its left extremity being the lower. The whole of the right posterior ventricular horn was in a condition of pap-like diffluence; its base communicated with the hole observed in getting out the brain. The left posterior ventricular horn was similarly but somewhat less affected. The diffluent fornix being scraped off the velum interpositum, that membrane was found to be entire and healthy. Commissura mollis had disappeared, and only a slight vestige of it remained adhering to the right thalamus, which was slightly the larger. The surface of both corpora striata and both thalami was softish; that of the left thalamus and right corpus striatum the more so. The inner substance of both thalami was soft, not normally distinct, and comparatively bloodless. The inner substance of the corpora striata appeared normal. There were scarcely any vascular fibrin-clots in the thalami, but numerous ones in the corpora striata. Cleft of the third ventricle of ordinary depth. The basic structures were generally covered by a yellowish, opaque, tough, laminated membrane. This fibrinous exudation extended under the arachnoid in stripes up the sides, and to the upper aspect of the hemispheres. It was most marked over the pons, and the quadrilateral space bounded by the optic commissure and the crura cerebri. On removing it, all the subjacent structures were found more or less changed. The tuber cinereum was soft and thin; the corpora albicantia were no longer white, nor their contours rounded and well-defined; on the contrary, they were of a dirty-gray colour, smaller than usual, nearly diffluent, and flocculent on the surface. The pituitary body was quite healthy. The crura cerebri were somewhat softer than usual. The fissura Sylvii and the mesian fissure, between the anterior lobes, were firmly agglutinated. The interior of the pons as usual the hardest, and the cerebellum as usual the softest, of the healthy encephalic structures. In getting out the brain, the lower extremity of the pons partially separated from the upper extremity of the medulla oblongata; the exposed structure appeared somewhat softened, as were likewise the walls of the fourth ventricles. The arteries were quite free from atheroma, and full of dark liquid blood.

Case XV.—J. J—, a farm labourer, æt. 38, married, from Fulham; admitted June 29th, 1854.

A darkish man of average frame and height, in tolerable health and condition. Expression fatuous, bewildered and unvarying, yet cunning. Eyes gray, pupils equal, sensitive. Tongue flabby, scarred. Pulse 64, so feeble it can with difficulty be felt. Sits stationary and semi-cataleptic. Forehead square, of fair breadth; sides of skull flat and high; vertex narrow. Head obscurely pyramidal. There is a long deeply indented scar, just to the right side of the middle of the sagittal suture.

He is stupid, bewildered, and answers the simplest question only after long hesitation, and usually incorrectly. He is in a condition of nearly complete dementia. His habits are dirty. He is stated to have " shown from childhood a dull morose habit and manner," but only to have become insane during " the last few weeks."

July 7th.—Habits are now clean. Though demented he is cheerful. Memory quite destroyed.

August 10th.—His physical condition and appearance have greatly improved.

13th.—At 1 p.m. was suddenly seized with complete hemiplegia dextra. An enema salis brought away a copious hard lumpy motion. At midnight all hemiplegic symptoms had entirely disappeared.

14th.—Up, and gentle as usual.

25th.—Since the seizure has been unusually cheerful, more restless, and less stupid.

September 20th.—Had a slight attack of hemiplegia dextra. An enema salis brought away a large quantity of small hard feculent lumps.

21st.—In his usual comfortable condition ; walking about, with no trace of his yesterday's seizure.

January 13th, 1855.—Continues semi-demented, restless, and bewildered. He is not morose, but taciturn, solitary, and capricious. In fair health and physical condition. At 4 p.m. had a paralytic attack. The right arm and leg were completely incapable of volitional motion, sensation and involuntary motion, the result of pinching, remaining. A salt injection brought away a copious scybalous motion. Pupils not unequal.

May 31st.—He gets more paralysed and his gait more devious and tottering. Has occasional palsy-shakes, always of the right side.

September.—During the early part of September was greatly enfeebled by an attack of that peculiar diarrhœa which is not uncommon among the paralysed. He never regained his strength after this, and was unable, from feebleness, to walk, or even stand.

18th.—Was seized with complete hemiplegia dextra. From

this date to the 15th October he was in bed, and nearly constantly convulsed on the right side. Mouth drawn to the right side. Sensation not abolished; pinching of the right arm sometimes made him move it, and sometimes produced cries and deprecating movements of the left arm. His cries during the night from the pain of the convulsions were often piercing. He incessantly ground his teeth, and produced a loud, grating, rhythmical, mill-like sound. During the convulsion the head was turned towards the right or convulsed side, by the convulsive action of the left sterno-cleido mastoid. This muscle on the left side was tense, on the right flaccid. No other muscle on the left side was spasmodically contracted.

October 20th.——Since the 15th has not been convulsed, the teeth-grinding has subsided, and he lies in bed with *both* his knees up. The right arm is completely motionless, but not insensible. He is sustained by liquid nutriment and custard pudding, and his bowels are rigorously regulated by salt enemata.

March, 1856.—Dementia continues. Since the last note he has been, when not under the influence of the convulsions, cheerful, and even merry. He would constantly grin and chuckle, smack his lips, and testify, by incessant uncouth gestures and grimaces, to the sensation of pleasure which pervaded him. Ghastly spectacles, and the groans of his fellow patients when in pain, seemed especially to excite in him pleasurable emotions. Thus, whenever he saw a corpse carried from the infirmary, he manifested, by pointing his finger and laughing at the passing coffin, the liveliest satisfaction; and the howling of a poor maniacal melancholic, makes him extremely jocular in feature and gesticulation. The teeth-grinding, grating, and rhythmical, has been nearly constant. The motion is always from left to right, and there is no back stroke of the lower jaw. The only distinguishable word he utters is too gross to mention. The right arm is paralysed but not insensible, and he can feebly move the right leg. Notwithstanding his constant dirty habits, he is quite free from sores.

June 28th.—He remains in precisely the same condition.

All his peculiar demonstrations of pleasurable emotion continue.

September 1st.—There is not the least change in his mental or bodily condition.

2d.—At 3 a.m. was found by the night-watch in a condition of convulsed coma. The convulsion was now exclusively of the *left arm and leg*. Coma and anæsthesia profound, except of the lower extremities. On tickling the soles no movements were elicited, but on hard pinching of the toes sufficiently evident movements of the leg resulted. The parallelism of the irides was maintained, but the movements of the eyeballs during the convulsions were always oblique. A salt injection brought away a copious lumpy motion. All the symptoms were unmitigated at noon. Left pupil the larger.

4th.—Coma profound. Convulsions of the left side continue. Anæsthesia of arms complete; movements of both legs, on pinching toes, sufficiently evident. Swallows with extreme difficulty. Rhonchus and mucous rattle in bronchi marked. Left pupil the larger.

5th.—No change, but that the convulsions are feebler. Slight rolling of the eyeball. At 11 p.m. the legs moved on the toes being pinched. Anæsthesia elsewhere profound.

6th.—Died at 2·30 a.m.

Autopsy.—Body not emaciated. Slight cadaveric stasis. Scalp thick and dense; on it, half an inch to the right of the middle of the sagittal suture, was a deep scar an inch in length. Scalp bloodless, except about the occiput, whither the blood had gravitated. Corresponding to the scar was a long shallow indentation in the right parietal bone, an inch and a half in length and of varying breadth, the greatest breadth being half an inch. The inner table of the skull was *not in the least* implicated in the depression. Skull thick and heavy; the sutures diaphanous and not hard to separate. The frontal bones were quite opaque, except at their mesian and transverse sutures. The parietal bones not quite everywhere opaque, but generally so. The temporal muscles very large and fleshy. The encephalon did *not* fill the skull. Dura mater thick, fibrous, wavy, *not* attached to cranial vault. Sinuses contained long, buff, fibrinous clots. Arachnoid normal, the usual paccionian adhesions along the sagittal suture alone existing. Sub-arachnoid serum most marked and equally diffused. The veins on the left hemisphere were very turgid with black blood; those on the surface of the right normally distended with ordinarily coloured venous blood. The hemispheres, while the brain remained *in situ*, were equal in size. On the removal of the brain, during which a large quantity of serum dribbled from underneath the arachnoid, the left hemisphere was evidently the smaller, and in it an obscure fluctuation was sufficiently perceptible. At the base of the brain the left middle lobe was markedly the smaller, and quaggy. On producing the centra ovalia, the left was found to be at least a third smaller than the right. While the medullary substance of the right centrum ovale pre-sented all the appearances and dimensions of health, the left was of a dirty buff colour, of toughish consistence, and of greatly diminished proportions, especially in its height. The left centrum looked in parts like a section of fine sponge, so large were its non-exuding puncta, most of which were empty, the rest accurately filled with dark fibrinous clots. The puncta of the right centrum were normal in number and size, but generally non-exuding and filled with clots. On laying open the lateral ventricles, the right was found everywhere quite normal; the left, particularly in its descending and posterior cornua, curiously changed. The posterior ventricular horn was dilated into a sac large enough to hold a small orange; its walls being greatly attenuated, and distended by limpid serum. The left descending cornu was shallow, broad, and filled with serum. The anterior horn was normal in size, and its walls of the usual thickness. The corpus callosum, fornix, septum lucidum, velum interpositum, corpora quadrige-mina, pineal body and its peduncles, were all *quite* healthy and well developed. The corpora striata were sym-metrical, of moderate size, and of natural consistence and appearance. The thalami were in the most marked degree unsymmetrical. The right, of natural size, presented a rounded outline and all the characteristics of health. The left, on the contrary, was shrivelled, collapsed, half the size of the right, and of a dirty-yellow colour. The posterior aspect of the ganglion was flattened, and especially implicated in this atrophy; it presented the appearance of shallow undulations. The left anterior thalamic eminence was still discernible and of healthy dimension. The commissura mollis was intact, but extremely soft. The inner structure of the left thalamus was composed of a dirty-yellow, here and there cribriform, bloodless, amorphous tissue, not soft or infiltrated. The section of the right thalamus discovered a perfectly healthy ganglion. The anterior and posterior commissures, both pillars of the fornix, and the antero-inferior region of the thalami, into which they are inserted, were all healthy in appearance, texture, and consistence.

Basic structures. All the cerebral arteries were quite black, and distended by dark liquid blood and long fibrinous clots. This appearance was universal. The arteries were free from atheroma. The tuber cinereum was extremely thin, the gray layer in front of and attached to the optic commissure, was in the same condition. The corpora albicantia were *not* symmetrical, the left being the smaller, much the softer, the more expanded and the less rounded. Its inner structure was softish and indistinct. The right corpus albicans was perfectly healthy. The left crus cerebri was a third smaller and much softer than the right, which was quite healthy. The pons varolii was remarkably small, otherwise normal. Medulla oblongata, anterior pyramids, olivary bodies, fourth ventricle, and cerebellum all healthy. Serum flowed from the spinal canal on dependance of the head.

Case XVI.—M. H—, æt. 47, labourer's wife, from Sussex; admitted May 30th, 1856.

A sallow, yellow-skinned woman, of middle height and average frame; emaciated, and in very feeble physical condition. Skin cool. Forehead transversely wrinkled; brows knit. Eyes gray; pupils unequal, right irregular, and the smaller; both are sensitive, the right much the less so

Nostrils markedly contracted at top of alæ. Upper lip deep, straight, nearly devoid of chiselling. Lips livid. Tongue very livid, tremulous, and slightly furred. Pulse 120, full. Brachial artery markedly rigid. Bowels, she says, open. Gait feeble. Has cough and dyspnœa, from chronic bronchitis. She constantly champs. Utterance distinct. Forehead broad, but not well shaped. Corona finely arched; sides of head, which is very long, markedly flattened. Memory is good, and she is not incoherent, when she can be induced to answer a question. This, however, is very difficult, as she is incessantly talking to herself in a melancholic strain; she imagines, among other horrors, that the world has come to an end, that all the inhabitants are murdered, and that "some of their heads are chopped off," &c. She iterates interjectional sentences after the manner of maniacal melancholics. This is a first attack of insanity, and is only of a week's date. While on the road to a new place, she heard that her mistress was very hard with her servants, and in the habit of discharging them without warning for trifling faults. This news appeared to distress and shock her. The day after her arrival at her employer's house, something went wrong in the churn, at which she was working. Apprehending, from what she had heard of her mistress's severity, that she was certain to be discharged, she became greatly agitated, and in a few hours was insane. Melancholia was the type of her first symptoms, which have progressed until they reached the maniacal pitch described above. Her father committed suicide, and his mother died insane. Liq. Opii, ʒss, in porter, h. s.

July 1st.—Had the draught at 10 p.m., yesterday. Slept till midnight, since which time she has been walking about the infirmary, bawling "murder," "fire," and shaking all the doors in the hope of escape. She takes no food unless forced to eat. Liq. Opii, ♏xl, in porter.

2d.—Quiet; but very depressed. Has been walking about all night, hallooing "fire," "murder," &c. Slept, while under the influence of the opiate, from 9 p.m. to midnight. Only takes food on compulsion. Right pupil markedly contracted, irregular, and horizontally flattened. Ext. Hyoscy., ʒss, h. s., instead of the opium.

3d.—Has had a perfectly quiet night, and is now calm. Takes solid food herself. Both pupils dilated by henbane; right, much the less so. Continue Ext. Hyoscy., ʒss, omni nocte.

4th.—Has had another good night, and takes food freely to-day. She trembles all over from the horror her delusions inspire. Pupils as yesterday.

5th.—Was walking about all last night, imagining every one was "to be ground up alive, consumed by fire," &c., Takes food fairly; lips tremble; teeth chatter. Right pupil still irregular, and markedly less dilatable by henbane than the left.

6th.—Has been crawling under the beds all night, and is now fearfully dejected. Eats well. Limbs tremble, and teeth chatter.

7th.—Is incessantly dressing and undressing herself; and has been crawling under the beds all night. Ext. Hyoscy., ʒss, bis die.

8th.—Has been crawling under the beds all night. She is now obstinately silent, and shuddering with horror. Right pupil as heretofore.

10th.—Has slept somewhat better; she kept in bed last night. Takes food fairly. She is now lying on the carpet; on being raised, she falls again a dead weight. This has occurred so many times that, while this condition lasts, she had better remain on the padded floor. Dyspnœa increases. Continue Ext. Hyoscy., ʒss, bis die. To be well sustained with milk, egg, and porter. The relation between the pupils is maintained, though both are dilated by henbane.

11th.—In bed, silent and wretched. Takes food with extreme reluctance. Oppression of chest increases. Pupils as heretofore. Continue Hyoscyamus. bis die.

12th.—Is much feebler; in bed. Silent; she trembles all over, and her teeth chatter. Takes food only on compulsion. Dyspnœa continues.

13th.—In the same pitiable condition. She is evidently sinking under the conjoint influence of pulmonary and cerebral disease.

14th.—Died at 10.40 a.m. Remained quite quiet till 4 a.m. Then commenced a loud moaning which lasted an hour. Took readily, during the night, what she was fed with, viz., milk, eggs, and brandy. Remained quiet till 8 a.m., when she was washed. Then clung to the attendant with great force, but was silent. After this she was calm, or at least quiet and still till 10.40 a.m., when she died of exhaustion.

Autopsy, twelve hours after death. — Body emaciated, though not markedly so. Rigor mortis slight in arms, more pronounced in lower extremities. Right pupil the smaller, and shaped as in life. Scalp thin, nearly bloodless, and easily torn down. Cranium of normal size and consistence, everywhere diaphanous. Sutures not ossified. Dura mater normally adherent to calvarium. Arachnoid healthy. The hemispheres are remarkably flattened, as if their substructures had given way extensively. There are few turgid veins in, and no serum between the pia mater and arachnoid. From the cerebral vessels exuded a copious liquid bright-red blood. Pia mater, of bright red colour, easily detached from convolutions; the latter were slightly redder than normal, of natural consistence, depth, and sinuosity. Centra ovalia appear larger than usual. Puncta of usual number and magnitnde, exuding a brightish red blood; there are, nevertheless, numerous linear red clots, which are more frequently met with towards the circumference of the hemispheres. Corpus callosum healthy. On laying open the lateral ventricles a curious scene of disorganization presented itself. The fornix soft, but not diffluent, rudimentary in size, but presenting somewhat of its natural outline, lay on the thalami, from which it was separated by *no* velum interpositum. The vertical part of the fornix was so soft that it could not be turned back with the corpus callosum. Pillars of the formix small, but otherwise normal. The corpora striata and thalami were all remarkably small. The corresponding bodies of opposite sides were equal. All these central ganglia were more or less soft;

their morbid consistence contrasting strongly with the healthy condition of the hemispherical ganglia. There was no commissura mollis, or any trace of it. All the structures forming the floor of the third ventricle were very soft and ruptured, so that cavity was quite patent below. The right corpus albicans was the smaller, softer, and not so white as its fellow. The right crus cerebri was ragged, markedly the smaller, and soft to diffluence. It appeared on the point of separating from the right thalamus and pons. The left crus was normal. The right thalamus contained less blood, and a few more empty channels than the left. The pons varolii was remarkably small, and perhaps softer than usual. It was, nevertheless, the hardest part of the encephalon. The cerebellum was as usual the softest *healthy* part of the encephalon. The medulla oblongata of normal hardness, but smaller than usual. The basic arteries were full of darkish blood; their coats of usual consistence. No specks of atheroma were discernible. The corpus callosum was not even on its superior aspect, owing to its substructures having softened, and given way. The third ventricle was completely open at the base of the brain, and the whole of its abnormally shallow cleft was thence distinctly visible; this condition of things being the result of the disappearance of all the structures, with the exception of the corpora albicanta contained in the quadrangular space, bounded anteriorly by the optic commissure and postero—laterally by the crura cerebri and upper edge of the pons varolii. In short, the tuber cinereum and substantia perforata having become softened to diffluence, had been dissolved in the subarachnoid or ventricular fluid. The fourth ventricle was normal.

CASE XVII.—A. M—, æt. 42, single, formerly a stock⁻broker, now a pauper; admitted April 10th, 1855, from the City of London Union.

A strong-framed man, of middle height, rather thin, in feeble health. Eyes hazel; pupils sensitive, equal. Tongue furred white, rather tremulous. Articulation very slightly affected. Nostrils equal. Gait feeble. Pulse 88, sharpish.

He is incoherent, full of mixed grand and horrible delusions, restless, and highly excited.

On the 1st of April he was apparently quite well.

On the 3d he was clearly insane, talking of an imaginary legacy of £1500, and calling himself the Marquis of Monteith. He is stated to have gone through an immense deal of trouble and anxiety, principally of a commercial character. He has tried, failed in, and abandoned various callings. He had just obtained a situation in the Commissariat, and was about shortly to embark for the Crimea, when he was overtaken by insanity. His habits are stated to have lately become intemperate. Ext. Hyoscy., Ðj, statim, et hora somni; Pil. Col. c. Cal., j, statim.

12th.—His intense excitement continues. He passes very restless nights in the padded room. Being under the domination of mixed grand and horrible delusions, he is walking about in the airing-court in a very irritable, morose, and dangeous condition. Hence an accurate account of his physical symptoms cannot be given. Continue Hyoscy.

13th.—Has torn up three blankets during the night, which he passed in the padded room, and against the door of which he was constantly hammering. To have the scruple of henbane in half a pint of porter, twice a day.

14th.—Very low to-day; refuses food, and says he has "a presentiment he shall be killed to-morrow." He is now quiet.

15th.—Fancies his food is poisoned, and that he is covered with vermin. To be fed with milk and eggs, and porter, as he refuses all solid food.

16th.—Tore up a blanket last night, and three blankets the night before. Has taken some strong beef tea and milk and eggs. He has a pint of porter daily, which, however, he can rarely be induced to drink. He refuses the henbane, and is very low mentally, but restless.

17th.—Intensely excited in padded room.

18th.—In padded room. He is much quieter, but highly destructive, constantly tearing up the blankets, &c. Just now he is on his knees in a fit of religious excitement. The pupils are contracted, somewhat irregular, and markedly sluggish. Has taken food more freely to-day than on any day since admission.

19th.—Continues so highly excited that he remains usually in the padded room.

20th.—High to-day; full of grand delusions; says he has "three millions of money," &c. Takes his food well. Bowels confined. Pupils are contracted and extremely sluggish. Pil. Col. c. Cal., statim.

21st.—Walking about in the airing-court in charge of an attendant. He is tranquil, but full of immense delusions; says he has "160 millions sterling" daily. He eats well. Pil. Hydrarg., gr. v, omni nocte. He sleeps in the padded room.

23d.—At 6.15 a.m. was quiet in bed. At 6.25 a.m. was got up by the attendant, and appeared much as usual. When on his feet, and about to change his wet shirt, he suddenly fell back insensible and convulsed. At 6.30 a.m. I found him comatose, with profound hemiplegia and anæsthesia sinistra. At 7 a.m. had a salt injection, which brought away a copious natural motion. At 1.30 p.m. the coma, hemiplegia and anæsthesia sinistra remained. The breathing is stertorous. He has had since his first seizure fifteen convulsed fits. In the intervals the eyes are open, and the left pupil is the larger. Repeat Enema Salis.

24th.—Since 8 p.m. yesterday the fits have been less frequent, and he has had none since 3 a.m. to-day. He has spoken a few monosyllables, and takes milk freely in tea-spoonfuls. His aspect is greatly improved. To have a quart of milk and eggs daily; repeat the salt injection. Hemiplegia sinistra continues.

25th.—Talks freely to-day, and takes liquid food readily.

26th.—Memory in abeyance. Unless the simplest question be kept constantly before him, he cannot answer it. He is regaining power over the left arm and leg; and though the leg recovers itself less rapidly than the arm, he has been able to walk a few paces. Sensation does not return so quickly as motion. He is becoming noisy; somewhat restless, and full of grand delusions. Pil. Hydrarg., gr. iij, bis die.

27th.—Memory is wonderfully better, and he talks comparatively rationally. Takes food well.

28th.—Full of horrible delusions; imagines the whole of London has been destroyed by fire, in consequence of the wickedness of its inhabitants. Uses his left arm freely. The memory is rapidly returning.

30th.—He is so extremely restless that he has been removed to the padded room to prevent him injuring himself, as he is incessantly getting in and out of bed, and, from his paralytic feebleness, falling and bruising himself.

May 1st.—Ext. Hyoscy., Əj, h. s.; continue Pil. Hydrarg., gr. iij, bis die.

2d.—He slept six hours soundly after the scruple of henbane. Ext. Hyoscy., ʒss, o. n.

3d.—Had a good night after the half-drachm of henbane.

4th.—Full of grand delusions. Had a good night. Ext. Hyoscy., Əij., h. s.; continue Pil. Hydrarg., gr. iij, bis die.

5th.—Face flushed. He is now extremely restless, but passed an excellent night. Continue pills and extract.

6th.—Full of melancholic delusions; imagines he " is poisoned by acetate of lead," &c. Has been very noisy, excited, and restless, from 2 a.m. till now (2 p.m.). Ext. Hyoscy., Əij, statim, et hora somni.

7th.—Has been quite calm since the exhibition of the sedative.

8th.—Being quite tranquil at 8 p.m. yesterday, he had not his usual sedative; in consequence of which omission he was, at 2 a.m., intensely excited and very violent. He then had Ext. Hyoscy., Əij, since which he has been perfectly calm. Tongue dry; face rather flushed. Continue Hyoscy., Əij, bis die.

11th. Mouth is getting sore. Pil. Hydrarg., gr. ij, o. n.; continue Ext., Əij, bis die. He is still excited.

12th.—Talking the completest incoherence of a large character in a solemn and sonorous tone.

14th.—In the infirmary, preaching to himself; imagines he is Christ.

15th.—Very depressed to-day; refuses food.

16th.——Has taken no food or physic for forty-eight hours. He is very morose and full of depressed fancies. This morning was very violent, seized an attendant by the scrotum, and, having taken out the side board of the bed, ran it through the window-panes.

18th.—Still very depressed; takes food sparingly and reluctantly; full of low delusions, fancying his food is poisoned, &c.

20th.—No better. Very destructive; staggering about airing-court. Omitte medicamenta.

22d.—Takes his food well; cheerful and talkative; calls himself the " Son of God."

23d.—Depressed and silent.

28th.—Imagines he has been poisoned.

29th.—Continues highly excited and destructive.

June 7th.——Very destructive and mischievous; grubs up the gravel, and throws it in or smears it on the other patients' faces.

August 4th.—Since last note he has been usually extremely irritable and morose, always destructive, mischievous, and collecting all manner of rubbish and filth. Since the 30th of May he has been nightly in the habit of defacing the walls of the single room, in which he sleeps, with stones, often sharpened. As he was stripped previous to going to bed, and his clothes removed, it was always a mystery how he got the stones. This morning the attendant, on removing his gutta percha chamber-pot, was struck by the singular weight of the utensil, which was half full of solid, natural-looking excrement. On examining it carefully, it was found to consist of stones and excrement in nearly equal proportions. He has been, in fact, in the habit of swallowing stones, and having passed them per anum, of using them to deface the extremely hard cement walls of his single room.

September 2d.—Has gradually become tranquil; his destructive habits have disappeared. He still, however, collects rubbish.

6th.—Says he has "800 millions a year, and all the railways belong to him." He is tranquil and orderly.

Both pupils are irregular, contracted, and very sluggish.

The large type of delusion, unaccompanied, however, by the least excitement, was maintained for about a month. Then he appeared quite free from delusion and coherent. When his former delusions were mentioned, he became irritable, and was evidently annoyed at the reminiscence. He remained in this tranquil and coherent condition till September, 1856. During the whole of this interval, though not incoherent, and apparently free from delusion, he was in a condition of incomplete dementia, his memory and the faculty of attention being greatly abridged. He was consequently unable to employ or amuse himself, and was usually somewhat bewildered, and rarely good-tempered. About the middle of September, 1856, an extraordinary delusion manifested itself. He now stated that the asylum was his property, and that he had bought it in the year 1206. On being asked how old he was, he stated his age to be about forty. He got over the discrepancy of the date of his imaginary purchase and of his rightly-stated age, by the delusion that he had existed from the foundation of the world; and that his body was renewed every 100 years by God, whose son, indeed, he imagined himself to be. During the twelve months ending September, 1856, his health and bodily condition were good, and the pupils were very contracted, irregular, and extremely sluggish. The habit of collecting rubbish never quite deserted him, though during the period of his tranquillity it dwindled into insignificance. He remained exactly in this condition till 1 p.m. on the 3d of October, when, immediately after dinner, he became suddenly convulsed and insensible. At 2 p.m. the coma was profound, paralysis and anæsthesia universal. The hardest pinching, or the most delicate tickling, produced no muscular response, whether of the irritated part, of the face, or larynx. During the convulsions, which were frequent and severe, the axes of the eyeballs, still parallel, were directed obliquely upwards, the left being external or diverging. The face and ears were very livid and hot, and a slight foam hung about the lips. The only conspicuous movements were those of the trachea, diaphragm, and pharynx, which was full of secretion. The breathing was entirely abdominal. The pulse was neither frequent nor feeble. A salt injection brought away a copious natural motion.

October 4th.—The symptoms have remained unchanged till 8·30 a.m. Now, for the first time, movements of the lower extremities are producible on tactual irritation. On tickling the soles, or pinching the toes, movements resulted, marked on the left side, slight on the right. The vigour of the movements is in direct proportion to the vivacity of the irritant; tickling produced trifling, pinching lively, motions of the legs. The face is evidently distorted into an expression of pain by hard pinching, while no such result followed tickling or moderate pinching. The eyes are glazed, the pupils not dilated. The breathing is laborious and not regular; the pulse is very feeble. Paralysis and coma complete. At 1 p.m. the symptoms are unchanged. At 2.30 he died.

Autopsy, twenty-two hours after death.—Rigor mortis not very marked anywhere, slightest in the arms. Cadaveric stasis most evident everywhere on the posterior aspect of body. Body in very good condition. Pupils contracted as in life. Scalp thick, dense, and full of blood. Skull thin, but hard, its inner table slightly eburnated, everywhere diaphanous. Temporal muscles immense. Dura mater and arachnoid quite normal. The pia mater very congested, of a livid red colour, its vessels distinct; it peeled easily off convolutions, which were of normal colour, depth, and sinuosity. The subarachnoid serum was copious, and the surface-vessels markedly distended and dark. The brain generally was small, but well proportioned. Centra ovalia equal, conspicuously studded with livid puncta, which exuded feebly on pressure. Linear red clots everywhere numerous in the medullary neurene; none in the gray substance. Corpus callosum very soft, but consistent, though subsequently nearly severed by the weight of the hemispheres. Fornix generally on the verge of diffluence; the body of the commissure could not be turned back from the velum interpositum entire; that membrane was markedly congested, but extremely well-developed. The septum lucidum was small, very soft, and in folds. The pillars of the fornix and the anterior commissure were diffluent externally, and flocculent. The commissura mollis had disappeared. The right thalamus was smaller, and much softer than the left. There was a rent an inch long at the junction of the right ganglion with the body of the right hemisphere. The sides of the rent were flocculent and soft, though not quite diffluent. It was doubtless produced in getting out the brain, which gave way at the point of least resistance. The left thalamus was much softer than normal, but less so than the right. The right corpus striatum was slightly smaller than the left. Both the great anterior ganglia were of normal consistence. All the structures at the base of the third ventricle were extremely soft, indistinct, and conglomerated from diffluence. Only one corpus albicans, the left, was recognisable. The pons varolii small, but of normal consistence. Crura cerebri very soft. These latter and the thalami were so much softened, that with a sweep of the finger they were removed clean, leaving the cornua ammonis and the pedes hippocampi perfectly exposed and intact. Medulla oblongata of normal hardness; cerebellum of normal softness : the former being the hardest, the latter the softest, part of the healthy encephalon. Arteries free from atheroma, but with thick coats and semi-patent ends.

Case XVIII.—L. K—, æt. 36, single, formerly a German merchant, now a pauper; admitted May 2d, 1855, from the City of London Union.

A fair, blue-eyed, thin-skinned man, above middle height, of average frame, tolerably well-nourished, in very feeble physical condition. Skin cool. Facial expression fatuous and unvarying, neither cheerful nor dejected. Pupils contracted, nearly insensible, but neither unequal or irregular. Nostrils equal. Upper lip tremulous, straight, its chiselling nearly obliterated. Utterance very imperfect and halting. Gait devious and straddling.

He is in an advanced stage of dementia, but is apparently free from delusion, and his spirits are unaffected. Though a Viennese, he can hardly remember a sentence of German. He is usually restless, but without purpose, and incoherently talkative.

He is stated to have been insane four months. The asserted cause is disappointed "hopes connected with business." There is a history of extravagance and of ruinous speculation. His father, who had frequently assisted him, at length got tired of doing so. He died last year, and bequeathed him nothing.

4th.—Excited and destructive. Tears up his blankets. Ext. Hyoscy., Əj, o. n.; Pil. Hydrarg., gr. v, o. n.

6th.— Continues very destructive, but in good spirits.

9th.—Much quieter.

14th.—Quiet, but incompletely demented.

20th.—Refuses his medicine. Omit it.

June 29th.—Has been since last note rather elated, but quite tractable. Habits are not destructive. Dementia does not advance. He is free from delusion apparently.

August 15th.—Always tractable, well disposed, and gay.

October 20th.—Tractable and well disposed. Extremely neat in his dress. He gets more demented, and is somewhat feebler. Tongue very tremulous. Left pupil usually slightly the larger.

March 1st, 1856.—During the last month has been usually very stupid and bewildered. He is to-day in bed very feeble and lost. He has occasional bursts of intense excitement, usually commencing in the evening. The left pupil is evidently the larger. He is rarely or never depressed.

June 28th.—Gets more feeble and lost. The pupils vary with the spirits; when elated and talkative, the left pupil is dilated wide; when depressed and taciturn, the pupils are equal, or nearly so, by the contraction of the left. The elated condition greatly predominates.

September 20th.—Gets more lost and feeble. The nocturnal accessions of excitement continue. He is labouring under the carbuncular diathesis. The left pupil has been always and markedly the larger during the last two months.

30th.—Having a large carbuncle over the sacrum, and being very feeble, he is kept in bed and on the water-pillow. Crucial incision of the carbuncle.

October 8th. —The sacral carbuncle is nearly healed, but the diathesis continues.

12th.—At 7 a.m. was found to be very stupid. At 9 a.m. he was in a condition of incomplete coma. Anæsthesia of the upper extremities nearly complete, of the feet much less so. The arms and legs are half flexed, and hard to straighten or flex completely. He appears as if in a condition of semi-convulsion. Pupils as heretofore; left dilated, right contracted. A salt injection brought away a natural motion.

13th.—The left arm and leg are paralysed and insensible.

14th.—He remains in a state of stupor, but is occasionally restless, and mumbling inarticulately to himself. He moves the right arm freely, the left is quite motionless, and insensible to the hardest pinching. The movements of the right arm and leg are very lively on their being pinched or tickled; those of the left leg on similar stimulation are, though sufficiently evident, much less lively.

15th.—In the same condition. Was extremely noisy last night.

16th.—No change.

17th.—Lies in bed with *both* his knees up. Left arm motionless, the right he moves freely; left pupil markedly the larger, and irregularly triangular, right pupil round and contracted; left arm and leg insensible to pinching or tickling.

21st.—Has had to-day two or three convulsions, confined to the left side.

22d.—The convulsions, which are of a few minutes' duration, and not preceded by any scream, continue at uncertain intervals, and are confined to the left facial muscles and the left labial angles.

23d.—The right half of the body is now convulsed, but the left conspicuously the more so.

24th.—Convulsions continue, but at longer intervals.

25th.—Has had twelve convulsions since last night.

During the seizures the left arm is violently extended and thrown up. He mumbles inarticulately to himself. Teeth clenched; swallows with difficulty. The paralytic symptoms, and anæsthesia of the left side, remain as heretofore.

26th.—Convulsions increase in length and severity; was in one from 9 till 11 a.m. In the intervals the right brow only is knit; left pupil as heretofore.

27th.—Convulsions continue.

28th.—Has had no seizure since yesterday at 5 p.m.

29th.—In articulo mortis apparently.

30th. — Moribund. Has had one short but severe convulsion. Right foot only moves freely on hard pinching; left foot insensible.

November 1st.—Has had three feeble convulsions up to noon.

2d.—Died at 9 p.m. Left pupil regular, but markedly the larger five minutes after death.

Autopsy, seventeen hours after death.—Body very emaciated. Left pupil, as in life, the larger. Rigor mortis distinct in both upper and lower extremities; more pronounced in the left arm and leg. Blood-stasis slight. Scalp tolerably thick ,not torn down very readily; from it exuded a good deal of darkish blood. Skull dense, but rather thin, everywhere diaphanous, except two or three square inches on either side of the sagittal paccionian depressions; these latter were *quite transparent* and very thin, but dense. The opaque patches in the parietal bones were the result of an unusual quantity of blood in the vessels of the diploe. A similar appearance existed, but in a less degree, in the right half of the frontal bone. Dura mater normally adherent to calvarium. An immense quantity of serum and blood escaped in getting out the brain. The reflected surface of the arachnoid, for three inches to the right of the superior longitudinal sinus, and in its whole length, was covered with a tough but congested layer of false membrane. On removing the fibrinous layer the arachnoid was found congested, and of a livid colour. The visceral arachnoid was everywhere healthy. Sub-arachnoid serum existed in enormously increased quantity. It formed large bullæ, and permanently distended the convolutions, especially on either side of the mesian cerebral cleft. The pia mater was congested and of a dull-red colour. The hemispherical ganglia were normal in colour and consistence, in depth and sinuosity of indentation. The centra ovalia presented fewer and less exuding puncta than normal; the substance of both was of natural consistence. The corpus callosum was well developed, and in every way healthy. The fornix, velum interpositum, commissura mollis, corpora striata, septum lucidum, corpora quadrigemina, the pineal body and its peduncles, were quite healthy. The thalami were markedly unsymmetrical, the left being flattened and devoid of its usual rounded prominences. Both ganglia were healthy in consistence, alike on their surface and in their substance; the surface of the *left*, however, had a remarkable buff-tint, and the section of its substance was manifestly the smaller. The contents of the inferior ventricular cornua were quite healthy, as were likewise the crura cerebri, the pons, the cerebellum, fourth ventricle and medulla oblongata; the lining membrane of the fourth ventricle was studded with small sudamina-like elevations. The corpora albicantia were equal, but small. The floor of the third ventricle was extremely thin, membraneous, and transparent. The horseshoe-shaped thinned gray substance in front of the optic commissure, and the tenuity of the tuber cinereum, were very conspicuous; through a rupture of this latter substance a large quantity of serum escaped. Arteries normal, not patent, and free from atheroma. The spinal canal was full of serum.

Case XIX.—J. B—, æt. 37, married, a fish-dealer, a pauper-patient from the City of London Union; admitted July 21st, 1856.

A tall fair man of average frame, emaciated, in feeble health and physical condition. Skin cool, complexion ruddy, expression neither depressed, cheerful, nor excited. Eyes blue; pupils contracted, unequal; left the larger, sensitive. In a darkened room the left expands freely, and is round and regular; the right remains contracted and nearly motionless. Upper lip long, straight, quite unchiselled. Mouth very broad. Tongue livid, large, tremulous; utterance slightly indistinct. Pulse 92, feeble, very compressible. Gait normal. He has a large superficial and healthy sore on the nates.

When admitted he was calm, and only partially incoherent. He imagined he was covered with lice.

He is stated to have been insane " two weeks ;" the ascribed cause is " excitement connected with betting." Originally in good business as a wholesale fishmonger, and owning several smacks, his business fell off in consequence of his addiction to the turf; he attended nearly all the races, and was an acquaintance of the notorious Palmer. At length, owing to the total neglect of his business, and to his losses on the turf, he became completely ruined. This climax is only of recent occurrence.

July 22d.—Full of horrible delusions, yet he is not depressed; talking of being poisoned by strychnia, &c. The contracted right pupil does not expand in the least in a dark room. Ext. Hyoscy., Əj, bis die.

23d.—He is intensely excited, and is just now quite naked in the padded room, having torn everything off himself. Ext. Hyoscy., ʒss, bis die.

25th.—In the padded room ; he has plastered himself all over with excrement. He is secluded because he has violently attacked another patient.

26th.—He has dirtied two padded rooms and torn up two blankets in the course of the night. He is now tranquil under the influence of Ext. Hyoscy., ʒss. He has taken food and medicine with extreme reluctance since his admission ; the only nutriment he takes freely is bread and water. He is compelled to take medicine, but he rarely takes the full dose.

27th.—Both pupils dilated by henbane; right the less dilated. He continues to strip himself. Continue Ext. Hyoscy., ʒss, bis die.

28th.—Still only takes bread and water readily ; refuses meat, and takes porter reluctantly. He is compelled to take milk and eggs.

August 1st.——Intense excitement continues. His delusions are principally horrible, yet he is not in the least depressed. He stands or lies on the floor of his single room all night, and makes the most hideous disturbance and howling conceivable ; takes food sparingly. Ext. Hyoscy., Ɔij, bis terve die.

7th.——Somewhat quieter under the influence of henbane. He imagines the head attendant is about to cut his throat, and requests a message to be sent to the Queen to prevent the murder. Sore on nates is well. Continue Ext. Hyoscy., Ɔij, bis terve die.

25th.——He has been much quieter since last note. To-day he is more excited.

28th.——Maniacal excitement continues; he strips himself. Continue Ext. Hyoscy.

September 2d.——Continues full of dreadful fancies, talking of strychnia and poisons. Takes food very sparingly. The right pupil continues contracted, feebly dilatable by henbane, and insensible to light.

3d.—Tranquil.

4th.——Full of mixed elated and depressed fancies, calls the patients all manner of singular nicknames, as Dr. Bartolo, Shakespeare, &c. He is extremely jocose.

9th.——He is sometimes intensely excited and violent for a minute or two, the next minute he is good-tempered and tractable. He is utterly incoherent and full of singular delusions, usually of a melancholic type, by which, however, he is not depressed. On September 5th he began taking Liq. Hyd. Bichloridi, ʒj, and Ext. Hyoscy., ʒss, bis die; on the 9th the extract was increased to two scruples.

October 23d.——Has continued the Ext. Hyoscy., Ɔij, and Liq. Hydrarg. Bichloridi, ʒj, twice a day from the 9th ult., with no apparent benefit. During this interval the short paroxysms of maniacal excitement have continued, but at longer intervals. The delusions have been of a mixed character ; he has been often very merry, and, what is singular, never depressed by his melancholic delusions. Notwithstanding his appetite has been excellent, and though he has taken all his diet, he has rapidly emaciated. Omitte medicamenta.

24th.—Good-tempered.

25th.—Emaciation advances, although he eats ravenously ; delusions horrible.

29th.—He gets so feeble and emaciated, that the recumbent is the only safe posture for him. To remain in bed
in Infirmary.

November 1st.—In bed, talking the most horrible ob-
scenity ; not depressed. He is utterly incoherent.

2d.—Has slight diarrhœa, under which, though it still
continued only slight, he sank in four days, dying of exhaustion on November 6th, at 2 p.m.

Autopsy. twenty-four hours after death.—Body emaciated.
Rigor mortis very slight; stasis trifling. Pupils rather contracted ; the right, as in life, the smaller. Scalp thin, easily
detached, bloodless. Skull thin, dense, nearly everywhere
diaphanous. On either side of the sagittal suture, and
just behind the coronal, there was a series of small
yellowish tuberosities of bone, smooth externally, of irregular outlines, and gradually merging into the inner
table ; at the seat of these bony eminences the calvarium
was not translucent. Dura mater healthy. Arachnoid
extensively adherent on the sagittal margin of both hemispheres ; the adhesions are composed of a tough, yellowish,
opaque substance. Arachnoid generally hazy ; sub-arachnoid serum very evident. The membrane over the quadrilateral space bounded by the optic nerves and commissure,
the crura cerebri, and pons varolii, is distended by serum.
On removing this serum all the structures were found more
or less softened, the greater softening existing on the left
side. Both crura cerebri, and corpora albicantia, were,
though still retaining their contour, most evidently softened ;
the left crus and corpus being manifestly the softer. In
tracing the middle cerebral artery through the fissura
Sylvii, the left descending ventricular cornu was, from its
extreme softness, laid open. The tuber cinereum was soft
to flocculence, and ruptured. The arteries quite normal
in structure, though too full of scarlet blood. Pia mater
healthy and not congested ; strips off convolutions with
tolerable ease. The convolutional neurine is nearly bloodless, and of an unusually dark-gray colour. Anfractuosities

of normal depth and sinuosity. Centra ovalia present a
usual number of exuding brightish puncta. Corpus callosum of healthy proportions, but rather softened. Fornix is
extremely soft; in attempting to raise it and turn it back,
the corpus callosum separated from it, nor could it be removed from the velum interpositum an entire lamina.
Velum interpositum well developed and healthy; at its apex
was a conspicuous yellow cyst, twice the size of the pineal
gland; its contents were small masses of cheesy matter
floating in serum. Commissura mollis none, nor any vestige
of it. Septum lucidum and anterior pillars of fornix
softened, but not diffluent; though not flocculent, their
contour was indistinct. The cleft of the third ventricle
gaping and shallow. The right corpus striatum and thalamus were evidently the smaller; the left thalamus being,
however, the softer, though not in a condition that ap-
proached diffluence; the left corpus striatum had the aspect
of comparative health. All these central ganglia were somewhat, though variously, softened; while the medullary and
cortical neurine of the hemispherical ganglia was of normal
consistence. Pons varolii, medulla oblongata, and cerebellum were healthy. The gray matter of the fourth ventricle
was superficially softened; the sides of the third ventricle
were composed of cerebral tissue, apparently healthy.

CASE XX.—S. B—, æt. 35, labourer's wife, from Sussex;
admitted April 4th, 1854.

A sallow, thin-skinned woman, of middle height, in fair
health and physical condition. Pupils dilated wide, equal,
round, but quite insensible. Tongue rather tremulous;
utterance indistinct. She is utterly demented, and incessantly talking incoherently. Jactitation and general excitement of manner and gesture are constantly present.

She is stated to have been insane many months, and to
have "had a fit a week before admission." No known
cause for her insanity.

From the day of her admission to that of her death, March,
1856, the patient's profound incoherent dementia lasted.
She was during these two years alternately in a condition
of maniacal elation and whimpering depression. When

elated, she frequently walked about for hours with a soldier's gait, and laughed, sang, or danced with frantic vehemence. In consequence of her noise and restlessness, she usually, when elated, slept in a padded room. When depressed she was less troublesome to her fellow-patients. She was now taciturn and stationary, and, though frequently whimpering, her depression was not otherwise demonstrative. If interfered with at any time, she soon became morose and violent; her language being at the same time horribly offensive and obscene. Towards the close of the case she rapidly emaciated, and, becoming gradually feebler, passed the last two months of her existence in bed. The alternations of depression and elation continued during this period. Death was preceded by some hours of profound unconvulsed coma.

Autopsy, twenty-six hours after death.—Skull thin, dense, translucent. Dura mater, arachnoid, and pia mater normal. The usual slight arachnoid adhesions existed at the sagittal margin of either hemisphere. Convolutions not deep, of normal colour and consistence. Centra ovalia large; puncta not numerous, small and livid. Corpus callosum and fornix healthy, except the anterior pillars of the latter, which were very and equally soft. Velum interpositum healthy. Anterior commissure soft. Corpora albicantia grayish and softened; the right the more so. The inner surfaces and bases of both thalami diffluent. The floor of the third ventricle in the same condition superficially. Commissura mollis thin, soft and flocculent. Crura cerebri softened, the right the more so; the most marked softening existed just where each optic nerve winds round the crus on its way to the bigeminal body. Tuber cinereum ruptured; ventricular serum flowed from the rent. Substantiæ perforatæ (anterior and posterior) on the verge of diffluence. Corpora striata healthy, equal; as were also the pons, cerebellum, and medulla oblongata. Sub-arachnoid, ventricular, and spinal serum abundant. Cerebral arteries full of blood, their coats healthy, ends not patent.

CASE XXI.—E. M—, private patient, æt. 64, widow of a tradesman; admitted December 24th, 1855.

A short woman of small frame, emaciated, in very feeble physical condition.   Facial expression nervous and apprehensive.   Face wan, parchmenty, not coloured, full of lines. Pupils very contracted, sluggish, right slightly the larger. Nostrils equal, expanded at their facial ends, contracted at the top of the alæ.   Upper lip broad, straight.   Jaws edentulous.   Tongue large, livid, slightly tremulous, with broad transverse rugæ.   Pulse 84, full; arteries markedly rigid and tortuous.   Gait very feeble.   Utterance normal.

She is extremely depressed, apprehensive, and nervous; owns she has had delusions of poisoning, but is just now free from delusion.   She is stated to be destructive of clothing, and to have recently attempted suicide.

She has been insane, or in the highest degree hypochondriacal, for about a year.   This is said to be a first attack, and its cause "family annoyances."

December 25th.—Ext. Hyoscy., gr. xv, h. s.   Slept well after the henbane for several hours, but became restless towards morning.

26th.—Ext. Hyoscy., gr. xxv, h. s.

27th.—The pupils are not dilated by the henbane; the right continues rather the larger.

January 3d, 1856.—From the day of her admission she has been very wretched, depressed, and hypochondriacal; often refuses food, from the delusion that she cannot swallow, and constantly imagines, or at least asserts, that it is impossible she can recover.

10th.—The hypochondriacal symptoms continue and increase; constantly complaining of some new unpleasant sensation, of hypogastric, cardiac, or lumbar pain; imagines she "is oppressed by water on the kidneys," that she "cannot swallow," &c.; takes only liquid food.

28th.—Since last note she has somewhat improved in appetite, aspect, and general condition; nevertheless she has been daily the subject of some new dysæsthesia; thus, sometimes she complained of abdominal distension or dysuria, then of diarrhœa, sometimes of dyspnœa, and often of dysphagia, &c.; constantly impressed with the idea that she is on the point of death.

April 25th.—No material change mentally, though her physical condition has greatly improved; often accuses her attendant of impossible cruelty, and sometimes swears she is covered with bruises, though on examination none are to be seen; to-day, imagines she is about to die from the exhalations of the fresh paint.

May 2d.—Telling the relatives of the other patients all manner of falsehoods regarding their treatment.

July 1st.—She gets more and more annoying to every one about her; she is incessantly whining over her own ailments, nagging at and telling lies of other people; sometimes asserts she has not passed water for six weeks, her bedclothes at the same time being wet with urine. The pupils remain as heretofore; health improves.

November 15th.—Has fewer hypochondriacal fancies, but gets more wretched. Her misery is now more demonstrative. She throws herself on the ground, strips herself, beats her head against the wall, and rubs any little wounds she may inflict on herself into sores. She is in fair health and condition; has taken food well during the last eight months.

21st.—Has acute bronchitis, under which, and refusal of food, she sank in thirteen days, dying on December 4th, 1856.

From the appearance of the first bronchial symptoms she constantly asserted she was dying, and sometimes, indeed, that she was dead. She frequently aggravated the dyspnœa, especially when she saw she was watched; and often refused food, imagining it was poisoned. Usually obstinately silent, she only spoke to whine over her misery and pain. The right pupil, during the last twelve days of life, was *markedly* dilated.

Autopsy, twelve hours after death.—Body somewhat emaciated. Rigor mortis slight, less in arms than legs. Pupils contracted, equal. Scalp thin, bloodless anteriorly, full of blood over the occiput, very easily detached. Skull of normal thickness, very dense, deeply marked with arterial channels; eburnated, not brittle; everywhere, but not equally, diaphanous. About the points of ossification in each frontal and each parietal bone the translucence was

less, from the presence of blood in the diploe.   Dura mater
normally adherent to calvarium.   Arachnoid healthy ; its
sagittal adhesions were more numerous and granular than
usual.   Subarachnoid serum slight.   Convolutions normal.
Pia mater congested, stripped off very easily.   Convolutional
neurine of a reddish-gray tinge, and containing some small
puncta, which, on pressure, exuded and became larger and
more numerous.   Centra ovalia markedly studded with large,
round puncta, patent, and, until pressed, empty ; on pressure
they exuded a thin livid blood.   Consistence of the cortical
and medullary neurine quite healthy.   Corpus callosum
healthy.   The vertical fibres connecting the lower surface
of the hard commissure with the fornix are thin and membraneous, but tough, and of the diaphaneity of thin horn.
The anterior pillars are healthy, the posterior somewhat
indurated.   The velum interpositum, pineal gland and
peduncles, anterior, soft, and posterior commissures, quite
healthy.   Corpora striata not very well developed; left
slightly the smaller.   Thalami are markedly unsymmetrical,
the right being about a fourth the smaller ; the diminution
is principally due to the disappearance of the postero-mesian
angle of the ganglion.   The anterior halves were equal
The internal structure of the thalami, the corpora quadrigemina, fourth ventricle, and medulla oblongata were
healthy.   The pons varolii somewhat smaller than usual ;
its structure quite distinct.   The corpora albicantia, tuber
cinereum, infundibulum, the subtantia and loci perforati,
were quite healthy.   The right crus cerebri was somewhat
flattened, but perfectly retained its fibrous structure.   There
was no softening in any part of the brain.   The arteries
were everywhere markedly atheromatous, and filled with
black soft clots.   The ends of the larger arterial subdivisions
were patent, and their coats much thicker and firmer than
normal.   The sinuses contained long, colourless, fibrinous
clots.   The brachial arterial was very rigid, firm, and thick ;
its cut ends ovally patent, its inner coat stained carmine.
This carmine staining was observable in the brain only at
the point or patch of atheroma.

CASE XXII.—J. J. W—, æt. 62, widower, a ruined stock-broker, a pauper patient; admitted October 4th, 1856.

A haggard, sallow old man, below middle height, of small frame, emaciated, and in a very feeble bodily condition. Facial expression fatuous and unvarying. Eyes gray; pupils irregular, markedly contracted, and very feebly sensitive. Nostrils expanded at their facial ends, the right ala markedly contracted at its upper edge. Upper lip straight, broadish, its chiselling obliterated. Upper jaw edentulous. Tongue immense, flabby, transversely corrugated. Pulse 92, not feeble; arteries rigid. Utterance rather halting; he jumbles the syllables of a very long word. He is not incoherent or depressed. Says he has lately been "rejected at Bethlehem Hospital, as they said he was paralysed." His memory is greatly impaired. He has been a stock-broker all his life, and has had the reputation of being wealthy. During the last few years his business has fallen off, and though main-taining a respectable appearance, he has been put to great shifts to maintain it. Since the death of his wife, his habits and manner, always odd, have become increasingly eccentric. He has only been recognised as insane during the last five or six weeks. His sister committed suicide.

October 5th.—He remained quite quiet till 7 a.m. to-day; then became restless and fearfully depressed, throwing himself on the floor, and beating it in anguish with his hands. He was in consequence placed in the padded room, where he re-mained till 7 a.m. on the 6th inst., when, having become calm, he was removed into the Infirmary. A scruple of Ext. Hyoscy., given at 8 p.m. on the 5th, greatly tranquillised him.

6th.—Continue henbane at bedtime; to have a pint of porter daily.

8th.—His nights, which from his restlessness are passed in the padded room, continue to be his most excited periods. Ext. Hyoscy., ℥ss, o. n.

9th.--He is cheerful for the first time since his admission.

10th.—Takes food with extreme reluctance, and in small quantities.

During the whole of October his symptoms remained of

the same type, but increased in intensity. Nearly always depressed, he was for many hours of every day in the lowest depth of mental agony. He now performed a kind of horrible pantomime of woe, wringing his hands, tearing his hair, and beating his head against the wall. His condition in fact was that of intense maniacal melancholia. He only took food on being fed, notwithstanding his appetite was tempted with custard, wine, and brandy. He took an inveterate dislike to his niece who had lived with and been very kind to him since his wife's death. He abused her when she came to see him, accusing her of all manner of crimes, including the having brought him into his present predicament.

All these symptoms continued and increased during November. His gleams of cheerfulness were rare and short. During the early part of the night he was nearly always maniacally excited, though he had half a drachm of extract of henbane every night at 8. After midnight he became quiet, and from 6 a.m. to noon was usually extremely drowsy. Even when not so, he sat motionless and silent. His obstinacy in regard of food continued, and was sometimes only to be surmounted by the use of the stomach-pump. When he talked, it was in that peculiar whining tone so affected by some preachers when "improving" a very lugubrious "occasion."

During December he rapidly emaciated, until indeed attenuation could hardly go further ; all his mental symptoms continuing as heretofore. On the 27th a crop of vesicles and bullæ appeared on both thighs. He was now from his extreme feebleness kept in bed. Gradually sinking, he expired of exhaustion at 6 a.m. on the 31st.

Autopsy, sixteen hours after death.—Body very emaciated. Rigor mortis well marked, as usual more evident in the legs than the arms. Pupils dilated, right the larger. Scalp very thin, easily detached, its vessels evident from the dark liquid blood they contained. Skull thin, everywhere translucent, dense, eburnated on both surfaces. Diploe not cancellous, and nearly bloodless. A good deal of livid blood dribbled from the saw-line. Dura mater rather more adherent to the vault than usual. In the right half of calvarium were four deep, quite transparent pits, all about an inch from the middle line; the first from before backwards, being placed in the lower third of the frontal bone, the second in the same bone just anterior to the sagittal suture, the third on the latter and extending backwards into the parietal bone, in which likewise the fourth pit was situated. Into the last three pits a deep channel, proceeding from the trunk-groove of the middle meningeal artery, ran. The third indentation was by far the largest, and contained the remains of cancelli. The least touch of the knife was sufficient to break the shell-like lamina which formed the vault of these erosions. In either temporal bone, the cavity of the tympanum could be laid open by a single sweep of a blunt knife; in the left, the superior semicircular canal, which by its prominence was very conspicuous, was similarly easy of exposure. Arachnoid healthy. It was, however, here and there opaque, opposite the dip of the convolutions. The usual Paccionian adhesions existed; they were markedly granular. Sub-arachnoid serum trifling. Pia mater not congested; it peeled readily off the convolutions, which were left quite clean. The cortical neurine had a slight tinge of red. Centra ovalia equal and normal. Their puncta few, large, and nearly all non-exuding. A few, by hard pressure of the circumjacent tissue, exuded feebly a livid blood. No puncta in cortical gray matter. Corpus callosum well developed, decidedly softened in its centre. The vertical fibres between the hard commissure and the body of the fornix diffluent. The fornix could not be removed in one layer from the velum interpositum, which was well developed, but nearly bloodless. Septum lucidum of not half its normal height, plicated, very soft. Commissura mollis none, nor any vestige of it. The thalami markedly unequal, the right at least a fourth the smaller—it was a third of an inch less broad than the left. A similar difference obtained between the corpora striata, but to a less extent. The substance of the right thalamus was much softer than that of the left; the section of the ganglia confirmed their external want of symmetry. The surface of the right corpus striatum was slightly softened. The substance of both these ganglia was natural in appearance and consistence. The whole of the lining membrane of the lateral ventricles was studded with minute, transparent, soft

vesicles, like sudamina. This appearance was limited by
the edge of the velum interpositum, none being found in the
third ventricle. The anterior and posterior commissures,
the corpora quadrigemina, the pineal body and its peduncles,
were normal. The cerebellum was, as usual, the softest
healthy part of the encephalon; the pons varolii being, as
usual, the hardest. This latter ganglion was of small size,
and its gray matter of a very pale tint. The medulla oblongata was small, but otherwise healthy. The crura cerebri,
corpora   albicantia,   and   substantia   perforata   posterior,
infundibulum, and pituitary body were quite normal. The
tuber cinereum was very thin, but not ruptured or soft. The
gray matter between the edge of the reflected corpus callosum
and the optic commissure was diminished to the thinnest
possible diaphanous lamina. The large cerebral arteries
were everywhere conspicuously studded with atheroma, by
which in many places the whole tube was encircled. The
smaller arteries, when not ostensibly atheromatous, were
extremely rigid and usually contained blood. The cut ends
of the internal carotids, the vertebrals, basilar, anterior,
middle, and posterior cerebrals were widely patent.

CASE XXIII.—G. W—, æt. 53, widower, a labourer, from
Herts; admitted May 7th, 1855.

A fair, short, weather-beaten man of small frame, emaciated, in very feeble health. Skin natural. Expression of
face vacant and, though he is incessantly talking, unvarying.
Eyes gray. Pupils unequal; right markedly the larger.
Tongue protruded slightly to the right. Utterance very
imperfect. Nostrils conspicuously contracted at the upper
edge of their alæ, right the more so. Upper lip broad and
straight, its chiselling effaced. Pulse 104, full, from
slight arterial rigidity. Gait feeble and tottery. He is
noisy, utterly incoherent, and incessantly talking. Stated
to have been insane twelve days. Beyond this, nothing is
known of his history.

May 8th.—Ext. Hyoscy., Əj, h. s.

10th.—Ext. Hyoscy., ʒss, omni nocte.

11th.—Ext. Hyoscy., ʒss, bis die.

14th.—Continue Ext., ʒss, bis die. Has been, from the

day of his admission, intensely excited, and usually talking with maniacal volubility and incoherence. He has, however, always been calmed by the henbane. To-day (the 14th inst.) he is much quieter.

20th.—Continues more or less excited, except when under the gentle influence of henbane.

June 25th.—Has gradually become quite tranquil. He is, however, demented. Omitte haustum.

October 20th.—This paralytic's delusions have been, when present, of a slightly melancholic type. He is, however, though always demented, at times free from delusion. He frequently imagines the walls are about to fall on him, in pursuance of which fancy he attempts to prop them up with his hands. The depressed mental condition is often expressed solely by his gestures, utterance being nearly suspended from advancing paralysis. His occasional maniacal excitement is subdued by seclusion in the padded room, and by ʒss Ext. Hyoscyami. The right pupil is always the larger, though not equally so. He is much feebler physically, and daily gets more demented.

March 1st, 1856.—The melancholic fancies have, during the last three months, disappeared, and the pupils have become equal. He is occasionally elated, when it is noticed the left pupil is the larger. His physical condition and utterance are considerably improved, and the dementia is less profound.

September 20th.—Has been apparently free from delusion since last note; but has gradually relapsed into nearly complete dementia, and into extreme physical feebleness.

February 4th, 1857.—Has remained in much the same condition till to-day, with the exception of a trifling diarrhœa of a week's duration ending 31st ult. He appears to have had a slight paralytic seizure during the night, the muscular power of the whole *left* side being manifestly diminished. He can with the greatest difficulty totter along. To be put to bed and to have a salt injection.

7th.—All the hemiplegic symptoms have disappeared, but he remains lost, and to the last degree feeble.

8th.—Semi-comatose and convulsed, especially on the *right* side, which is paralysed, but not deprived of sensation.

When the right arm or leg is pinched, he moves not the irritated, but the opposite limb. Enema Salis.

9th.—Much better; speaks in monosyllables when roused. Has had no convulsion since yesternight. He moves the right arm when it is pinched, but not the right leg, on irritating which he moves the left arm.

February 11th.—Hemiplegia dextra continues. He is speechless and semi-comatose, but not convulsed.

13th.—Right arm and leg volitionly motionless. No convulsion except of the right leg, which often twitches. When the right leg is pinched, he does not move *it*, but the left arm or leg. Swallows with great difficulty.

14th.—Died at 11·30 a.m.

Autopsy, five and a half hours after death.—Body in good condition. Right pupil the larger. Scalp not bloodless nor congested, stript off easily. Skull dense, not thick, diaphanous. Diploe mottled with patches of slight congestion, which were nevertheless obscurely translucent. Dura mater normally adherent to calvarium. A nearly transparent Paccionion pit existed in the left parietal bone, opposite the centre of the sagittal suture. Arachnoid not adherent, except slightly along sagittal margin of both hemispheres. Sub-arachnoid serum *most* copious. Visceral arachnoid generally rather hazy. Surface-veins gorged. On the surface of the centre of the left hemisphere, commencing about an inch from its sagittal margin, was a dusky-red ecchymosis of the pia mater, two inches long by about an inch wide. Corresponding with this, on removing the pia mater, was found a largish irregular cavity, the walls of which were composed of ragged, semi-diffluent, mixed red and white, convolutional neurine. A similar but less advanced and smaller cavity existed on the mesian surface of right posterior lobe. Pia mater easily stript off convolutions, which had a slightly wrinkled appearance. Puncta of cortical substance exuding and numerous; of medullary substance few, of largish calibre, and very feebly exuding. Corpus callosum normal. Callo-fornal fibres degenerated into a peculiar membranous layer, of the appearance and translucence of thin horn; this lamina was rather tough and extended into the septum lucidum. The body of the fornix remained entire after the removal of this extensile vertical layer. Pillars of fornix small, not soft or flocculent. Anterior commissure, velum interpositum, pineal body, posterior commissure, and corpora quadrigemina normal. Commissura mollis none, nor any vestige of it. Thalami *very small* externally, equal, not so white as usual. The substance of both is quite healthy. Corpora striata healthy, but small. Cleft of the third ventricle shallow, and, on the removal of the velum interpositum, gaping. All the ventricles distended by serum. Tuber cinereum membranous in tenuity and translucence, not soft or ruptured. Corpora albicantia small, but white and normal in consistence. Pons varolii, cerebellum, medulla oblongata, crura cerebri, quite healthy. Arteries thicker, less translucent and collapsible than natural; full of dark blood and clots, here and there specked with atheroma. Root of each petrous bone slightly cancellous.

CASE XXIV.—H. C——, æt. 56, widower, a physician; admitted January 24th, 1856.

A short well-made man of average frame and in good physical condition. Facial expression vacant, neither elated nor depressed. Eyes gray; pupils equal, not round, irregular, contracted, and very feebly sensitive. Nostrils expanded at their facial apertures, contracted at top of alæ; the right appears slightly the more contracted. Upper lip long, straight, unchiselled; mouth immensely broad. Tongue large, livid, rather tremulous. Teeth not ground down. Pulse 80, feeble; arteries apparently not rigid. Gait feeble, not devious. Utterance rather indistinct, from the imperfect articulation of double consonants and the confusion of the syllables of long words.

He is cheerful and full of singular delusions, all of a more or less exalted type; says the asylum belongs to him, and that he bought it two months ago for £1500, and that he expects " to be sent for by the Government in consequence of a speech on the war he made in his own room to an audience of twenty." He is partially incoherent, and his memory is greatly impaired.

He is stated to have been quite well till "last Good Friday," when he had an attack of hemiplegia *sinistra*. From this he recovered in a week, and was then able to resume his professional avocations. The present attack of insanity is of a month's duration, and dates from a second attack of hemiplegia sinistra.

There is a history of long domestic unhappiness. His only child, two years since, went to Australia. He has never written to his father, who has been deeply pained by the seeming neglect.

February 27th.— Full of curious large delusions; imagines he is about to be created an earl, that he is the "Master of the Horse," and that he is on the point of "starting for Margate in a carriage-and-four."

June 27th.—His large delusions have been since last note mixed with extraordinary melancholic fancies. Imagines a lately discharged patient "drugs and debauches every woman he approaches," and that his son has shot this imaginary libertine with a rifle-ball. He is often at night intensely excited, morose, violent, and destructive.

September 23d.—His mixed delusions continue. He gets more irritable.

January 1st, 1857.—Gets more lost mentally, and is usually taciturn, bewildered, and stationary. When roused he is very irritable and accuses those about him of theft; calls his medical attendant "a damned scoundrel," imagining he has stolen his watch, and threatens, without any provocation, to "knock down" the other patients and "put them in strait-jackets."

February 6th.—Remains in the same mental condition. At 7 p.m., while in bed, was seized with convulsions, confined to the *right* side; paralysis, coma, and anæsthesia being at the same time universal and profound. Never rallying, he expired at 1 a.m. on the 7th of February.

Autopsy, seventeen hours after death.—Body fat and in excellent condition. Pupils rather contracted, equal, not round. Scalp easily detached; bloodless except about occiput. Skull of normal thickness and density, nearly everywhere diaphanous. Here and there a trifling diploïc congestion diminished, though it did not destroy, this translucence. The arterial channels were somewhat the deeper on the left side; some of the upper channels ran into a long, shallow, narrow depression, nearly transparent, just to the left of the anterior third of the sagittal suture. The bases of the anterior aspect of both temporal bones were conspicuously cancellous. A touch of the chisel immediately laid open the tympana and what appeared to be an immense exaggeration of the mastoid cells. Dura mater normally adherent to calvarium. Arachnoid healthy. Subarachnoid serum abundant. Pia mater of natural colour, and stripped easily off convolutions, which were healthy. Puncta largish, feebly exuding, mostly filled with red linear clots, more rarely empty and non-exuding. Corpus callosum normal. Callo-fornal fibres and septum lucidum diffluent. Fornix small, soft, with difficulty retroverted entire. Velum interpositum small. Right corpus striatum and thalamus conspicuously the smaller. The surface of the former not rounded, quaggy. The postero-internal angle of the latter not salient, but rounded off. Left corpus striatum quaggy, but less so than the right. Left thalamus normal except in size, which is manifestly below par. Its posterior angle markedly more salient than the corresponding right angle. Commissura mollis healthy. Crura cerebri soft externally, right the softer. Tuber cinereum normal, not soft, but ruptured. Corpora albicantia small, not naturally white; of normal consistence. Pons varolii normal; its right half is perhaps rather the softer. Cerebellum and medulla oblongata healthy. Arteries everywhere atheromatous, with patent ends, many varicosities, and usually distended by blood. The sinuses contained immense red and buff fibrinous clots.

CASE XXV.—J. K—, æt. 54, a butler, married, the father of several children; admitted September 16th, 1856.

A tall, well-made, slim man, thin and in feeble health. Skin cool. Facial expression neither elated nor depressed, unvarying. Eyes hazel; pupils equal, contracted, and very sluggish. Nostrils equal. Upper lip broad; its chiselling effaced. Tongue large, clean, rather livid. Teeth not ground down. Pulse 92, fullish from rigidity of the arteries, which are not tortuous. Gait natural. Speech not quite distinct; he lingers over and jumbles the consonants of a long word. Complains of pain in the occiput, which, he says, keeps him awake at night. He is not incoherent just now, but owns that he has lately laboured under the most singular delusions, *e. g.*, that he " swallowed himself and brought himself up again," that he " saw himself rolled up into a huge snowball," and that he imagined, without the least foundation for the story, that his wife had been lately " brought to bed." Good tempered, cheerful, and tractable.

He is stated to have been insane " about two months." The attributed cause is grief at the death of a favorite daughter, ten months since. He has been full of all manner of absurd schemes for some time past, and " has lately spent a large sum of money at Brighton, or rather had ordered a large amount of useless goods, the delivery of which was stopped by his friends."

17th.—Restless, talkative, joyously excited, and full of schemes. Says he is " going to take a party of eighteen gentlemen from the asylum over the Continent, himself acting as courier, and receiving, besides board and free passage for himself, a franc a day from each traveller." Liq. Hyoscy. ʒj, h. s.[1]

18th.—Liq. Hyoscy. ♏lxxx, h. s.

21st.—Liq. Hyoscy. ♏lxxx; Liq. Hyd. Bichloridi, ʒj, bis die, which he took regularly till the 10th of November.

Up to the 5th of November the type of the delusions and his general mental condition remained the same. He was incessantly restless, except when tranquillised by the henbane, talkative, full of foolish projects, elated, partially incoherent, and quite inconsecutive in ideas and action. Towards the end of October this mental condition, though still sufficiently perceptible, gradually declined, his physical state at the same time daily becoming feebler. The contracted pupils were dilated equally by the henbane. By the 5th of November every vestige of joyous excitement

---

[1] ʒj Liq. Hyoscy. contains the active principles of ʒss of the extract.

had vanished. He was now depressed and taciturn. Says he has "abused his master's confidence."

November 6th.—Imagines he is about to be hanged.

7th.—Imagines he has committed every conceivable crime, including murder, adultery, sodomy and bestiality; he is fearfully depressed.

29th.—He continued in precisely this condition till 7 a.m. to-day. He was now found in epileptiform convulsions; of these he had in six hours eighteen distinct attacks; during the intervals the coma, anæsthesia, and paralysis were profound and universal. Salt enemata elicited copious natural stools.

30th.—Has had no convulsions since yesterday. The arms remain very rigid. Has uttered a monosyllable or two. Swallows liquids freely.

December 1st.—Talks intelligibly, but incoherently. No vestige of paralysis or anæsthesia remains.

2d.—Sitting up; depressed and feeble.

January 30th, 1857.—Has been since last note taciturn, never speaking unless spoken to, stationary, reluctant to take food, and very depressed. He has never smiled, and if questioned regarding his horrible fancies, repeats with minute detail of circumstance, time, place, and person, the whole repulsive catalogue. He is much feebler. To be removed to infirmary.

February 4th.—Has evidently had a slight seizure of hemiplegia dextra. The right elbow is strongly flexed, and he cannot raise the arm from the shoulder. The right leg drags. Speech and gait markedly halting. He is pale, emaciated, and feeble. To go to bed. Enema salis.

5th.—Remained sensible till 9 a.m., when he suddenly became comatose, and was attacked with convulsions of the right arm and leg. He had several convulsive seizures of the right side during the day, between which hemiplegia dextra and coma remained complete. Gradually sinking; he died at 10 p.m.

Autopsy, forty-two hours after death.—Pupils rather dilated, equal. Rigor mortis slight in the upper, marked in the lower, extremities. Scalp bloodless, except over

occiput. Skull hard, not thick. Diploe congested. Inner
table highly glazed, mottled with numerous small arbores-
cent, livid vessels. In the left parietal bone, half an inch
from the sagittal suture, and an inch from the confluence of
the coronal and sagittal sutures, was a conspicuous, nearly
transparent, deep concavity, of the size of a horse-bean. A
similar but smaller pit existed in the left frontal bone, just
anterior to the coronal suture, and in the same line with
the larger depression; into both these an arterial channel
ran and ended. In the right frontal bone, an inch from
the mesian line and from the superciliary ridge, a deep,
abrupt depression, into which no channel ran, existed. The
whole skull, from the congestion of the diploe, was less diaphanous than usual. The bases of the petrous portions of
both temporal bones were markedly cancellous. Dura
mater normally adherent to calvarium. Opposed surfaces of
arachnoid not attached, except slightly along the sagittal
margin of the hemispheres. Visceral arachnoid rather
hazy generally. Subarachnoid serum copious. Through
the arachnoid were here and there discernible bright-red
patches of the pia mater; these were more conspicuous on
the right side. Pia mater stripped off readily, and was of
a natural redness. Convolutions of normal depth and
sinuosity; from their gray matter, which had an evident
reddish tinge, no puncta were elicited even on hard pressure. Right centrum ovale much the smaller. Puncta of
medullary matter of normal number and size, very feebly
exuding even on hard pressure; everywhere pervaded by
red linear clots. No serum in ventricles. Corpus callosum normal. Callo-fornal fibres diffluent. Body of fornix
small, very soft. Septum lucidum not half its usual
height, semi-diffluent. Left corpus striatum markedly the
smaller, very soft, its surface not rounded, but undulated.
No tenia semicircularis on the left side. Right corpus
striatum of normal size, but not of natural rounded contour.
Right tænia semicircularis very evident. Sections of the
corpora show the right to be at least a third the larger.
The surface of the right is rather quaggy. Both anterior
pillars of the fornix soft to diffluence. Anterior commis-

sure very soft, markedly oblique, the left extremity being the lower. Commissura mollis none, nor any vestige of it. Both thalami *very small*, left the smaller. The inner and posterior part of the left no longer angular but rounded; the corresponding right angle being well defined. Anterior thalamic eminences normally distinct. Surfaces of both thalami softish, not flocculent; their substances, especially that of the left, soft. The section of the left confirms the appearance of its external inferiority in size. All the basic structures contained between the optic commissure, tractus, and upper edge of the pons, very soft, including the tuber cinereum, corpora albicantia, and substantia perforata posterior. Both inferior middle lobes soft, left markedly the softer. Left crus cerebri and left half of the pons much the softer, the right crus and right half of the pons not being of natural hardness. Medulla oblongata the hardest, cerebellum the softest, of the healthy encephalic structures. Arteries not atheromatous, but having much thicker coats and more patent ends than ordinary.

CASE XXVI.—A. T——, æt. 54, single, of no occupation; admitted May 16th, 1855.

A tall, fair woman, of large frame, emaciated, and in feeble physical condition. Skin cool. Cheeks florid from the separate injection of the venules. Eyes gray; pupils unequal, right the larger, both contracted and sluggish. Right eyeball the more uncovered, which gives to it a fallacious appearance of prominence. Ptosis sinistra. Upper lip long, straight, devoid of chiselling. Pulse 78, full from rigidity of the artery, which is not tortuous. Tongue largish, furred white, tremulous, transversely rugose. Gait feeble. Utterance natural. She is not incoherent, but extremely depressed; the memory is greatly impaired.

Her brother, with whom she lived as housekeeper, and to whom she was deeply attached, died some months since; and though reckoned a man well to do in the world, his estate was found to be insolvent. Since his death, by which event she was left destitute, she has been noticed to be very eccentric; during the last three weeks she has been recognised as insane.

17th.—Continues depressed. She is usually coherent and well disposed. Has curious hypochondriacal fancies; imagines she passes no urine, and that, if she continues to take fluids, she will become "full of water and burst."

19th.—Says she is "full up to the throat," and imagines her bowels are confined. Ol. Croton gtt. j, statim.

21st.—Though the bowels are known to have been well opened, she still complains of constipation and of the sensation of fulness.

July 17th.—Has remained very depressed since last note, though her dejection varies in degree. When very low she is full of horrible fancies, imagining she is the devil, that her throat is too small for deglutition, that her intestines are "blocked up," &c. At these periods she takes food with extreme reluctance, and in small quantities. She is physically feebler.

20th.—Gets more wretched; refuses food and medicine, and insists on walking about the infirmary without shoes or stockings. This condition continuing unmitigated up to the 23d, she was injected by the stomach-pump on the four days ending that day with a pint and a half of milk, three eggs, three ounces of brandy, and ɱl Liq. Opii.

On the 24th, she took liquid food naturally, after the exhibition of the stomach-pump.

27th.—She is much less depressed and feeble.

October 9th.—Has been comparatively tranquil and cheerful since last note, though in the interval she has had a severe attack of erysipelas of the legs. She sometimes even grimly smiles. During the present week she has taken to pick herself, and imagines she has no tongue. If addressed, replies—"It's no good talking to me, I've got no tongue, and I can't speak." She takes food reluctantly, and has unquiet nights. Liq. Opii, ɱxl, o. n.

December 21st.—Has remained depressed since last note, and has often been very annoying from her impulsively obscene, morose, and abusive language. The pupils have remained since her admission contracted and nearly insensible, the right being usually the larger.

June 12th, 1856.—She continues depressed and taciturn. Without any assignable reason, will often say to any one who may be talking, " Oh, what a damned lie," " Hold your tongue, you damned fool," and more frequently uses interjectional obscene abuse, too gross to repeat.

December 20th.—Her moroseness, depression, and singular abuse, have continued. She is much feebler.

February 10th, 1857.—Gradually sinking, she expired of exhaustion, after a semi-conscious, motionless, silent stupor of thirty-six hours' duration, during which, by clenching her teeth and constricting the fauces, she obstinately refused food. These were her only voluntary movements.

Autopsy, twenty-four hours after death.—Body very emaciated. Pupils dilated, right the larger. Scalp thin, bloodless, easily detached. Skull thin, diaphanous, dense, brittle. Diploe anæmic. Dura mater normally adherent to calvarium; its sinuses contained a few buff clots. Opposed surfaces of arachnoid quite free, except at the sagittal margins of both hemispheres. Visceral arachnoid rather hazy, but nowhere opaque. Subarachnoid serum copious. Pia mater rather congested. The gray cortical substance has a tinge of buff. On pressure, numerous puncta are developed in it. Puncta of the medullary substance of normal number, size, and efflux. Corpus callosum healthy. Fornix, velum interpositum, and septum lucidum, all small, but otherwise healthy. Corpora striata and thalami externally equal; the former paler than usual, the latter of a dirty white colour, and markedly dwindled. The internal substance of the thalami was healthy; a vertical section showed that the *right* ganglion was *much less deep* than the left. Commissura mollis intact, very thin. Cleft of the third ventricle *extremely shallow*. Tuber cinereum very thin, not ruptured, though of membranous tenuity and translucence. The loci perforati, in front of the optic commissure, were similarly circumstanced. Corpora albicantia small, else healthy. Crura cerebri less fibrous and hard, especially the right, than usual. Pons varolii very small, else normal. Medulla oblongata, fourth ventricle, and cerebellum, normal. The ventricles were distended by serum, which likewise flowed copiously from the spinal canal. All the arteries were *distended* by black blood ; the tubes were much firmer, less collapsible, and less translucent than natural. The internal carotid markedly patent, and slightly specked with atheroma. Brachial artery was rather rigid, and had patent uncontractile ends.

CHAPTER VI.

An analysis of the pathological appearances of these twenty-six cases discloses as its most remarkable features —1st. An uniformity of the unaffected cerebral structures. 2dly. A nearly undeviating regularity in the implicated ganglia and commissures; though the degree and nature of implication varies in almost every case— varies, in fact, according to the intensity of the symptoms, the stage of the disease, and the mode of death.

And first, of the unscathed encephalic structures. In order fully to comprehend and utilise the pathology of any psychical disease, the appearances of the complicated congeries of vesicular and tubular masses called the brain (the function of each of which is to the mind as different as that of lungs, liver or kidneys to the body) should be classified, with the hope of eliminating from the analysis all the healthy or quasi-healthy structures, so that the little light emitted from it may be concentrated on the organs most or really affected.

In the observations about to be made on the apparently unaffected encephalic ganglia of general paralysis, there is no intention of implying that they are actually not implicated in the lesions so recognisable in other parts of the brain, but rather that their damage is so slight as to be difficult or doubtful of recognition, even to the practised eye. That all the psychical ganglia are more or less affected is evident enough from the profound dementia which, inter alia, is the inevitable destiny of those in whom the malady runs out to its *natural conclusion*. On the other hand, the *progress* of the disease, while it shows that towards its close the declension of pure intellect is its most noticeable mental symptom, and that therefore the hemispherical ganglia are then profoundly affected, likewise indicates that, often in the earlier stages of the malady, the emotion of pleasure or pain alone is morbidly exalted, and therefore as yet only the thalami [1] are implicated.

Supposing, as we have a right to suppose, the proportion between the lesions witnessed after death and the intensity of the symptoms during life to be *the same in all the encephalic ganglia*, there are certainly many which, though the function ascribed to each of them is manifestly no longer naturally performed, appear, as far as the unaided senses go, wholly or comparatively un-

---

[1] From the fact that all cerebral acts are, or may be, followed by a painful or pleasurable sensation, from the anguish which the histories of general paralysis constantly disclose, and from the revelations of early unreported autopsies, I have been gradually led to the conclusion, that, as the thalami are the original seat of the disease, so they are likewise the centres in which arise all sensations of pleasure or pain, whencesoever derived, whether the result of sensuous, intellectual, or moral stimulation. As moral acts are, in the majority of minds, by far the most frequent causes of keen pleasure or pain, it is not surprising that the parent ganglia of these emanations should be especially influenced by moral emotions, and that in extreme cases of protracted agony (and perhaps ecstasy), they should be overpowered and become disorganised. According to these views, the appropriate designation of these great central ganglia should be thalami pathemici. Though the whole chain of facts and reasoning, by which I have arrived at these results, is too lengthy and controversial to be admitted into a volume which professes to be a practical account of general paralysis, I may, perhaps, hope to find, at some future time, an opportunity for its publication, and so to make known my views regarding the physiology of the disease.

affected; thus, while the central parts of the encephalon, the thalami, commissura mollis, fornix, septum lucidum, corpora albicantia, &c., are more or less palpably softened, or in some way changed, the convolutions, pons varolii, medulla oblongata, cerebellum, &c., have all or most of the appearances of health. It may indeed be that the organic changes capable of producing momentous and persistent *intellectual* aberrations are, from the extreme functional delicacy of the hemispherical vesicles, so slight, as entirely to baffle the unaided eye; while in the grosser seats of the will or emotions marked functional deviation cannot be accompanied by irrecognisable lesion. As, however, this marvellous touchiness of function is more than we have a right to presuppose, it is reasonable to conclude, on comparing the mental symptoms and pathological appearances, that the disease, commencing in the seat of the emotions in the central parts of the brain, spreads gradually to other ganglia, to the seat of the will, the corpora striata, or to the seat of the intellect, the hemispherical ganglia; but that these and other similar masses are not sufficiently damaged for the recognition of their real structural lesion. On the other hand, it may be (and certainly in the earlier stages of the malady often is) that the peripheral neurine—the seat of the intellect—is only *functionally* affected from the structurally changed central ganglia; that no morbid appearance is detectable in the hemispherical ganglia, notwithstanding their marked functional deviations, simply because they have undergone no histic change, they being only functionally irritated from the degenerated or disorganised thalami. From a review, then, of its pathology, I think it will be evident that, as the post-mortem appearances of general paralysis are good indices of the degree and order of lesion in the several affected ganglia, so the insignificance or negation of such appearances, in instances of morbid increase of the function attributed to the slightly involved or quite unscathed ganglia, indicates the secondary nature and distant origin of these periphero-cerebral emanations.

The encephalic ganglia, which in general paralysis are found to be unscathed, or but slightly affected, are, as I have before mentioned, principally those placed in the periphery of the viscus. They are the hemispherical ganglia, usually both in their convolutional and medullary neurine, the pituitary body and infundibulum, the pons varolii, medulla oblongata, and cerebellum; to these may be added the skull and membranes. The cerebral organs, which are but little affected, are the corpus callosum, the corpora quadrigemina, the pineal body, the corpora striata, and posterior commissure. In reviewing the slightly varying appearances of these structures in the twenty-six autopsies, a record of which I have preserved, each structure will be mentioned separately, and from the periphery towards the centre.

And first, *of the cranium and membranes*. The skull is usually healthy. Nearly always of natural thickness and translucence, it is generally dense in texture, but not brittle. In patients who have died of exhaustion, and whose bodies are very much emaciated, the scalp is thin, exsanguine, and easily detached; in these cases the skull is, as just described, thin, translucent, dense, and bloodless. In examples of the malady which do not go on to their natural termination in exhaustion, and in which the patient is still in a tolerably good bodily condition, when the supervention of convulsions, bronchitis, or diarrhœa, brings the case prematurely to a close, the scalp is often gorged with blood, and especially so in its occipital region, from cadaveric stasis. Accompanying this condition of scalp is often found a congested diploe, which renders the transmission of light through the skull sometimes impossible, and always imperfect. At the sutures, however, where the cancellous structure is trifling, the more usual diaphaneity is maintained.

In two of the three cases in which the cranium was unlike what I have just described, it was immensely thickened and heavy, quite opaque, very dense, and eburnated on the surface of both tables, nearly all cancellous appearance being at the same time obliterated from diploe. The skull was in some parts half an inch thick. In the third case (XV) the calvarium was everywhere opaque, except at the sutures. In Cases XIII and XV, there were good reasons for supposing that old injury of the skull was at least an adjuvant of the malady; in the one case (XIII) the patient having suffered a severe cerebral concussion, immediately followed by facial paralysis, two years before the supervention of insanity, and four years and a half before death; and in the other (XV) a deep indentation, corresponding to a scalp scar, being found in the outer table of one parietal bone. Of the history of the third case (XII) nothing was known, not even so much as her name.

In several cases, a very singular appearance presented itself in the petrous portions of the temporal bones; these, the hardest bones in the body, had undergone a cancellous degeneration, so that the cavity of the tympanum could be laid open with a single and feeble stroke of a blunt knife, and the whole length of the superior semicircular canal by a sweep of a similar instrument.

In most instances of thin and diaphanous calvaria, there are usually unsymmetrical erosions in the cranial vault, which are often *quite transparent*, so that small print can be easily read through them. These have been regarded as resulting from the pressure of enlarged paccionian bodies. Occasionally similar pits have been found, where none of these bodies exist, namely, on the inner table of the frontal bone, within an inch of the superciliary ridge. In these latter cases, therefore, absorption of the bone cannot be ascribed to the pressure of these peculiar masses. Indeed, it may be fairly doubted whether any of these depressions are the result of paccionian enlargement, as usually I have found no gland whatever corresponding to the pit, and never one sufficiently large to account for its size and depth. Frequently the depressions, which are most common in the parietal bone, are out of the paccionian range, they being usually found an inch or more from the sagittal suture. What likewise contributes to throw doubt on their heretofore assumed causation is the presence of a large vascular channel, which enters their outer side, and which nearly always terminates there. Is it possible that varicosities of the middle meningeal artery are their real cause?

THE MEMBRANES.

The *dura mater* is never structurally changed. Rarely firmly attached to the cranial vault, it is usually indeed detached from it. Occasionally the detachment is complete, a manifest vacuity existing between the calvarium and the upper surface of the fibrous envelope. In these cases the membrane is no longer tense, but limp and in folds, abundant subarachnoid serum being always found associated with this plicated condition of the dura mater.

The appearances of the arachnoid are very regular. Its opposed surfaces are usually quite free from adhesion, except along the margins of the great superior longitudinal cleft. Here adhesions are found in nearly every case. Usually trifling and merely marginal (being apparently only slight exaggerations of the normal paccionian adhesions), they are now and then more extensive; even in these rare instances they are confined to a square inch or two on either side of the superior longitudinal sinus. The adhesions, whether extensive or insignificant, are *invariably old*. Usually white, membranous, and yielding, they are occasionally yellow, granular, and tough. The visceral arachnoid is often found distended by subjacent serum, which is sometimes present in sufficiently large quantity to raise that membrane here and there into bullæ. This condition is only found in instances of sudden coma, and is usually found associated with the above-mentioned plicated dura mater. The arachnoid covering the basic quadrangular space, bounded by the optic commissure and tracts, the crura cerebri, and pons varolii, is occasionally thickened, and often distended by serum. This distension is always associated with ruptured floor of the third ventricle, a remarkable and frequent appearance, which, though I once regarded as cadaveric, I am now inclined to consider as happening during life. In only one instance (Case XIV) did the serous envelope appear markedly and recently changed; and even in this instance the tough, laminated, fibrinous membrane covering the basic structures was rather under than in the arachnoid, a peculiarity which was especially manifest at the sides of the brain, round which long, thin strips of similar membrane wound, and here and there attained the upper aspect of the hemispheres. These strips, which shone through the arachnoid, could be easily separated from it, and thus disclosed themselves lying between it and the pia mater.

Pia mater.—The condition of the immediately investing membrane of the encephalon presents but little uniformity of appearance. This discrepancy is owing to the patients' various modes of death, and to their then different bodily conditions. In the more recent cases the sanguiferous tunic was markedly congested and of a bright or livid-red colour. In those who died of exhaustion, it was usually pale and nearly exsanguine; while in those whose death was preceded by more or less marked or long convulsions, it was found of every variety of colour, from anæmic paleness to bright or livid redness. This variety of colour and congestion was owing to the more or less complete manner in which the pia mater had relieved itself by serous effusion. In no case whatever was any fibrinous exudation or other product of inflammation apparent on the pia mater, except in the remarkable case (XIV) above mentioned. The pia mater usually strips readily off the convolutions, and especially so in the cases complicated with arterial atheroma. There is always a general resemblance between the condition of the pia mater and of the velum interpositum and choroid plexuses.

The Hemispheres.—The changes in the gray substance of the hemispherical ganglia are neither many nor striking. Usually, indeed, the seat of the intellect presents all the appearances of health. More rarely,

and in protracted cases of profound dementia, the convolutions are somewhat flattened, and their anfractuosities less deep and sinuous than normal. The texture of
the gray neurine is sometimes soddened, and to its gray
colour is now and then added a marked buff tinge. The
flattened, dilated, and infiltrated condition of the convolutions is doubtless traceable to the pressure, thrust,
and imbibition of a morbidly copious subarachnoid serum.
The paucity and shallowness of the sulci are probably
congenital; their buff tinge the result, perhaps, of degeneracy. It was to be anticipated that the colour and
blood-condition of the convolutional gray matter would
be similar to that of its immediate hæmal investment.
Accordingly, we find in the rare instances where the pia
mater is congested, and of a bright-red colour, the hemispherical gray matter has an evident red tinge, and a
few exuding red puncta distributed through its substance.
Usually, however, it is bloodless, and few or no puncta
are detectable—a condition which is but little changed
by pressure. When the gray substance has been
softened or soddened by the circumjacent serum, the
pia mater does not strip off clean or easily; on
the other hand, when the vessels of the pia mater par-
take of the atheromatous condition frequently so evident
in the primary branches of the Willisian circle, the
membrane strips off readily and quite clean. At the
bottom of the sulci, where the vascular supply would
appear principally to enter the cerebral periphery, the
foramina of the torn, rigid vessels are, though bloodless,
large and patent.

The *pons varolii, medulla oblongata, cerebellum, the
inter-cerebral commissure or processus è cerebello ad
testes, the fourth ventricle and its walls, the corpora*

quadrigemina, the pineal gland, its peduncles, and the posterior commissure, are nearly always in their natural condition. The pons is nearly invariably the hardest, and the cerebellum the softest, part of the *healthy* encephalon. This peculiarity of the latter organ is probably owing to the cadàveric stasis of serum into, as the body lies on the occipital protuberance, the most depending part of the cranial cavity. The medulla oblongata usually partakes, to a modified extent, of the hardness of the pons. In one case, the pons and medulla separated, in getting out the brain, at the transverse line which divides them; but as the examination was not made till seventy-two hours after death, not much importance can be attached to this, perhaps cadaveric, softening. A somewhat similar though less marked softening existed in Case XIV, the autopsy of which took place twenty hours after death. This is the exceptional case so conspicuous from the presence of the laminated fibrinous membrane, the product of inflammation, which covered all the organs at the base of the brain.

As the connecting link between the unaffected, or but slightly changed, peripheral structures and those central organs which are found to be profoundly affected, I now approach the morbid changes discernible in that immense commissural apparatus which forms the great bulk of the brain, viz., *the white matter of the hemispheres.* This intermediate mention is their due, as much from pathological condition as from anatomical site; for by their more discernible lesions, as compared with the trifling or invisible changes of the true peripheral organs, and by their slighter or less conspicuous damage when compared with that so evident in the central ganglia, they hold the same mid-state as, in site and function, they hold to these structures. The most remarkable change met with in the condition of the white hemispherical fibres, is a want of symmetry in the opposite masses. This condition can sometimes, though rarely, be made out before the production of the centra ovalia, that is, before each hemispherical ganglion is sliced down to the level of the corpus callosum. One hemisphere, while they are yet intact, appears slightly the smaller. It is only, however, on the production of the centra ovalia that the want of symmetry is, from its conspicuousness, certain. The smaller centrum ovale, a diminution attributable to atrophy, is always on the same side as the more affected thalamus. The colour of these fibres is seldom changed. In the solitary instance (Case XV) of this change that has occurred to me, the commissural fibres of the left and smaller hemisphere were markedly tinged buff, and contrasted conspicuously with the pure white of the opposite mass. Whenever this change of colour exists, it doubtless, as in this instance, corresponds in side with the more implicated thalamus.

The consistence and texture of the white hemispherical fibres are rarely changed from their ordinary dough-like state of cohesion and uncleanness of fracture. The only exception to this rule occurred in Case XV, in which these fibres were markedly tough, and nearly of sponge-like consistence and arrangement. I have never found these masses of fibres softened. That circumstance, however, in which the bulk of the medullary fibres of general paralysis principally differs from its condition in healthy subjects, is the state of the vascular puncta, the peculiarities of the cut ends of its vessels. It is natural to these great masses to present, on hori-

zontal section, a fair number of small and round exuding
red points. Now, in the subjects of our malady, all
these conditions are in the same brain often found
altered. Usually diminished in number, but increased
in size, they are irregularly angular, and feebly or
not at all exuding, the colour of the exudation being
dark or livid red. All these peculiarities are often remarkable in one centrum ovale, the other presenting no
apparent deviation from health. When this unsymmetrical state of the puncta exists, the centrum containing
the morbid appearances is always found to correspond
in side with the more implicated thalamus. In the
more recent cases the puncta are usually numerous,
round, exuding, and brightish red; in chronic cases, or
where the patient is cut off by some intercurrent
exhausting disease, the puncta, though exuding, are
rarely bright. Irregularity in their outline is always
associated with atheromatous, or, at least, imperfectly
elastic cerebral arteries. Nor is this mere coincidence;
it is doubtless cause and effect. The cut ends of the
arteries are irregularly angular or patent, because their
coats are feebly and unequally contractile, or rigid and
no longer resilient. That this explanation is not forced
is proved by the fact that, where the atheromatous
arteries are the more conspicuous, there likewise the
foramina are larger and more irregular; and where, in
the same brain, the atheroma is unequally distributed in
the principal vessels of the opposite hemispheres, there
also, associated with the greater morbid deposit, are
found more markedly irregular and patent puncta. In
the instances where the puncta, though full, are non-
exuding, the arteries are blocked up with soft, livid-red,
or hard, pale-buff, fibrinous clots; often the puncta do

not exude, because the tubes leading to them are permanently empty and cut off from the circulation. The former condition is sometimes found when the paralytic has been suddenly carried off, while still unexhausted, by coma; the latter condition usually only obtaining in those cases where marked arterial atheroma or rigidity is discoverable after death in the brain.

Having thus disposed of the unaffected or slightly affected cerebral structures of general paralysis, and cleared the way for the consideration of the more deeply implicated ganglia and commissures, I will indicate the boundaries of that space in which these conspicuous but varying changes are always to be found. Bounded above and in mid-front by the corpus callosum; postero-laterally and towards the front by the mesian edge of hemispherical medullary fibres; inferiorly and from before backwards by the reflected layer of the corpus callosum, by the loci perforati, the optic commissure and tracts, the tuber cinereum, corpora albicantia, substantia perforata posterior, and the crura cerebri; and posteriorly by the tubercula quadrigemina, the pineal body, and upper edge of the pons varolii, is a space containing the following organs or structures (from before backwards): the corpora striata, the septum lucidum, the anterior commissure, the pillars and body of the fornix, the velum interpositum and plexus choroides, the thalami, soft commissure and posterior pillars of the fornix, the eminences in the inferior and posterior ventricular horns, the posterior commissure, and the pineal peduncles.

Some of the organs forming the boundaries of this space usually, and always many of the organs in it, are in the brains of general paralytics found markedly changed. As in very severe cases most of these structures are evidently involved, and as the great and constant implication of the thalami and of their appendages, the fornix, soft commissure, the floor of the third ventricle, and the crura cerebri, point unmistakeably to these exactly central structures as the focus or original seat of the malady, I shall, reversing the order hitherto pursued in tracing its pathology (from the circumference towards the centre of the brain) proceed at once to state the marked deviations from health which are so recognisable in these central structures, and to trace, by the lesions of the adjacent organs, its progress, direction, and extent.

The thalami.—It appears that, in twenty-three out of twenty-six cases, there were discernible in one or both thalami sufficiently marked, though varying, morbid changes. In the three cases in which they are stated to have been normal, the thalami, though equal and of natural consistence, were much diminished in size; though their power of assimilation remained, its vigour had become greatly impaired; they were, in fact, in an advanced stage of atrophy. It has, indeed, never been my good fortune to see, in the same case of general paralysis, two equal and well-developed thalami, though I have not seldom seen *one* of healthy structure and dimension.

The thalamic changes in these twenty-three cases vary, whether in degree, kind, or site, in nearly every instance. One or other thalamus is diffluent or softened, or both are similarly or profoundly affected. One thalamus is degenerated, but not softened, the normal structure being replaced by a yellow, toughish tissue, the opposite ganglion having all the appearance of health. Sometimes, though rarely, without any evidence of disorganization, and with none of pravity but an anæmic condition, the inner structure of one thalamus is found grooved with long empty channels, apparently vascular. This bloodless channelled condition is usually very conspicuous in one thalamus, the other presenting numerous exuding puncta, and no empty grooves.

The changes in the thalami of general paralytics may, I think, be referred to one of four conditions: 1st, to disorganization or softening; 2dly, to degeneracy with or without induration; 3dly, to atrophy, diminution of size without apparent histic change; 4thly, to vascular changes without any recognisable structural lesion, to hyperæmia with numerous exuding puncta, to anæmia with many empty channels. The arrangement of the analysis is made entirely according to the commonness and gravity of the morbid changes, and is probably in many instances exactly the reverse of the order of their occurrence.

And first, *of softening or disorganization of one or both thalami.* Under this head will be included every variety of diminished thalamic cohesion, from slight though perfectly appreciable softening, through the gradations of marked softening and semi-diffluence, to the complete breaking down and disintegration of the ganglia. Of the 26 cases, in 11 there was observable well-marked softening; of these, in 3 (Cases XI, XVII, XX) instances, one of the ganglia, or some part of it, was quite diffluent and broken down; in 3 (Cases III, XIV, XVI), one or both were on the verge of diffluence, and had a greatly diminished sharpness of outline; and in 5 (Cases I, XII, XIX, XXII, XXV), though softened, their condition did not approach that of diffluence, and their contour remained naturally well defined. In 4 (Cases I, III, XII, XXII), only one ganglia was affected; in 7 (Cases XI, XIV, XVI, XVII, XIX, XX, XXV), both participated, though usually not equally, in the lesion. Diffluence of the whole ganglion, or of both ganglia, is rare; it is commonly confined to the surface of one thalamus, to its base, to its anterior aspect about the insertion of the pillars of the fornix, or to its point of junction with the edge of the hemispherical medullary fibres. When the surface is quite disorganized, the thalamus is no longer smooth, but ragged, flocculent, and of a dirty buff-red colour. This appearance is not uncommon on the opposite sides of the cleft of the third ventricle. When the base of a thalamus is diffluent, the diminished volume and lower plane of the more affected organ render the lesion very conspicuous. In instances of pronounced thalamic diffluence the commissura mollis is broken down; it has entirely disappeared, or what remains of it hangs in shreds from one ganglion.

The organs are sometimes semi-diffluent. Their shape is now slightly changed, their outline being less sharp and well defined than usual. Though the surface is not flocculent, it speedily becomes so when subjected to the ordeal of a small and feeble stream of water, under which the ganglion rapidly disintegrates.

But softening, without any change of form in the ganglia, and unaccompanied by diffluence or by rapid dissolution under the stream, is doubtless the most common form of thalamic lesion of cohesion recognisable to the unaided eye. The structure of one thalamus is palpably much softer than its fellow or than the adjacent hemispherical structures, the declining coherence being usually accompanied by diminished volume, by bloodlessness and confusion of the inner structure of the ganglion. The difference in the condition of the vessels on the surface of the affected or more affected ganglion, and on its adjacent corpus striatum, often indicates which is the more profoundly implicated. On the ganglia of one side the natural colour, the minuteness of subdivision, and the number of the vascular ramifications, at once stamp the organs as healthy; while the entire absence of vessels on the other side, or their pallor, paucity, and coarseness, as evidently point to the site of the lesion.

The mental symptoms coincident with thalamic softening are, whatever their type, of an intense character. The vehemence of the more aggravated cases of paralytic maniacal exaltation or melancholia it would be difficult to exaggerate. The gradation of intensity is clearly in proportion to the more or less advanced softening. With the more marked mental symptoms are found diffluent thalami; the lesser grades of maniacal elation or frantic melancholy being coincident with semi-diffluent or merely softened ganglia.

And secondly, *of degeneracy of the thalami*. This condition is less frequently noticed than the former, and may or may not be accompanied by induration. It is always associated with diminished volume. The degenerated thalamus (where, as usually happens, only one is affected) at once asserts its pravity by its conspicuous atrophy, its yellowish colour, and sometimes by its shrivelled look. These appearances in two cases (XVIII and XXVI) were confined to the surface, in another (XV) they pervaded the entire structure of the ganglion. Of the two cases (VIII and XXIII) I have witnessed of symmetrical degeneracy, in one (VIII) the ganglia were singularly small, hard, and very dark internally; in the other they were very small and dirty white internally. In only one case (XXIII) of degenerated thalami was the commissura mollis broken down. It is, on the contrary, usually firm, even to induration, and well developed. The mental or maniacal symptoms accompanying this condition of thalami are less intense than those associated with softening, while the dementia of degeneracy is the more profound, and usually the more protracted. All the cases terminated in sudden convulsed coma of some days', and in one instance (Case XVIII) of some weeks' duration, the result, in every instance, of immense serous effusion in the sub-arachnoid and ventricular cavities.

Thirdly, of *simple atrophy of the thalami*, without apparent change of structure. In 9 cases there was simple atrophy of one or other, or both thalami. In one instance (Case II) the left, and in 4 (Cases IX, XIII, XXI, XXIV), the right was markedly the smaller, without any recognisable structural change. In 4 instances (Cases IV, V, VII, X), both thalami were much and equally diminished in volume. Though of some of the instances of thalamic atrophy I have preserved no record of their vascular condition, I have little doubt that in all the cases of equal atrophy the ganglia were bloodless, or nearly so; and that, in the five instances of unsymmetrical atrophy, while the larger ganglion presented the appearance of vascular normality, the smaller or atrophied organ was anæmic and probably deeply grooved with empty blood-channels. In Case X the thalami were atrophied equally, but the right ganglion was bloodless and channelled, the left retaining much of its healthy appearance. In Case XIII the whole encephalon, including both thalami, was everywhere and equally studded with numerous non-exuding clot-puncta. In Case IX the right and atrophied thalamus was bloodless, the vessels on its surface being at the same time few, pale, and small.

The mental symptoms associated with atrophy of both thalami, though absolutely remarkable, are, relatively to the intense psychical symptoms of thalamic softening, insignificant. Of the nine cases of thalamic atrophy, only one (Case IX) emulated the intensity of the symptoms attending ganglionic softening. In this instance atrophy was confined to the right organ.

The remaining section of the analysis is that in which the only recognisable lesion is vascular. Of this variety I have only one instance to adduce, and that is one of the most remarkable cases I have ever seen. A criminal lunatic (Case VI), after forty-one days of culminating morose mania, died, having been only a fortnight resident in the asylum. During the whole of that period the symptoms of maniacal melancholia were of the most intense character, the right pupil being at the same time insensible, irregular, and contracted. After death (by exhaustion) the thalami were found smaller and much darker internally than usual, both having large puncta and blood-channels in their interior. The right was a fourth the larger. From the history of the case, its rapid progress, its intensity of moroseness, and the coincidence of the right pupillary affection, I am inclined to regard this as an instance (according to my present knowledge a solitary instance) in which the patient was hurried off while the thalamus was yet in an incipient condition of passive congestion, and in which the hyperæmia of the more affected ganglion was demonstrated by its tumefaction.

I have now to consider the *relation of the site of the thalamic change to the mental symptoms of the disease.*

From the coincidence of affected right pupil with mental depression, and of affected left pupil with elation, I draw the conclusion that the ganglia of pleasure and pain are on different sides of the encephalon. A chain of reasoning, of which these facts are the premises, and the revelations of early autopsies, have led me to the further conclusions—1st, that the right thalamus is the ganglion of natural painful, and the left thalamus that of healthy pleasurable, emotion ; 2dly, that the marked melancholic and elated mania, so characteristic of general paralysis, are the results of morbid changes respectively in the right and left thalamus ; and 3dly, that disease of these great central ganglia is to be regarded as the primary physical cause of the malady, as the focus whence disorganization or degeneracy spreads to the adjacent ganglia and com- missures.

The results of 26 cerebral autopsies are remarkably favorable to these opinions. Of 9 cases of intense un- mixed paralytic melancholia, in 7 instances the right thalamus was markedly diminished in size ; and in 4 of these 7 it was either diffluent or much softened.

Of the 2 remaining cases, the shortest that have ever occurred to me, being respectively of forty-one and twenty-two days' duration, in 1, the latter, the thalami were equal, and both much softened with diffluence of the commissura mollis, of the *right* crus cerebri, and of the *right* corpus albicans, the left corresponding structures being unaffected ; and in the other the right thalamus was the larger (the whole brain being at the same time much congested), evidently from its greater hyperæmia.

Of the 4 cases of maniacal elation, or of grand delu- sion, in all the left thalamus was found to be the smaller, and either degenerated or softened.

Of 8 cases of alternating melancholic and elated mania, or of mixed or alternating grand and depressed delusions, in 5 both thalami were softened, in 2 they were small (in one of these latter the equal ganglia were indurated), and in the remaining case no other unusual thalamic appearance presented itself than marked diminution of the right ganglion. Of these 8 cases, in 5 the right, in 1 the left, thalamus was the smaller, and in the remaining 2 the ganglia were equal.

In 5 examples of profound dementia, accompanied by no, or very slight, delusion, but in 2 of which the alternation of elation and depression, though not remarkable, was sufficiently evident, the thalami were equal and very small.

On comparing this classification of the mental symptoms with the thalamic pathology of general paralysis, it appears that the post-mortem condition of the thalami and the adjacent ganglia, in all the instances of pure paralytic melancholia, directly confirms the opinion of the thalamic origin of the disease, and distinctly points to the right ganglion as the especial seat of its depressed variety. Though in one instance of maniacal morose melancholia the right thalamus was the larger, in all the other instances, diminution of size being taken as the principal criterion of ganglionic implication, I do not regard this variation as contradictory of the hypothesis. The patient in this case, of only forty-one days' duration from the first insane symptom to his death, perished before the usual atrophy which succeeds passive hyperæmia had set in, and while the ganglion was still tumid from primary congestion. In the other rapid case, of twenty-two days' duration, though the right thalamus was not the more affected, the equal ganglia being small and much softened with destruction of the commissura mollis, the *right* crus cerebri and *right* corpus albicans were nearly diffluent. In both these instances of intense and rapidly fatal paralytic melancholia the right pupil was contracted and nearly insensible, the left iris being in every respect normal.

The relative condition of the thalami in the 4 instances of unmixed paralytic elation is directly confirmatory of the thalamic origin of the disease, and of the hypothesis that implication of the left ganglion is the cause of maniacal exaltation.

In the 5 cases of profound dementia associated with no, or very slight, delusion, the equally atrophied thalami at once suggest the idea that the function of the dwindled emotional ganglia, they no longer containing vesicles sufficiently healthy to be stimulated by the ideas or perceptions to demonstrations of pleasure or pain, had for ever lapsed, and that, therefore, to complete dementia was added profound or comparative apathy.

The condition of the emotional ganglia in the 8 instances of mixed or alternating grand and depressed delusions, or of melancholic and elated mania, while it endorses the opinion of the thalamic origin of the malady, hardly affords so direct a confirmation of the theory of emotional localization as the other groups of the classification. In 7 of the 8 cases both thalami were changed, either by softening, induration, or atrophy. In the remaining case (XIII), not a strongly-marked specimen, psychically, of the malady, the right thalamus was the smaller, with absorption of the commissura mollis and softening of both inferior middle lobes, probably attaining or influencing the bases of the thalami. The implication of *both* ganglia in these mixed or alternating cases therefore clearly confirms the theory; as it demonstrates the necessity of structural change in both emotional ganglia for the production of the mixed form of the mental symptoms. On the other hand, with the diminution of the right thalamus, which occurred in 4 of the 7 instances, in 2 it does not appear that the maniacal melancholia, though frequently of the intensest order, exceeded, or endured longer than, the maniacal elation; while in Case XXIII, in which the left thalamus was the smaller, the elated period of the four earlier months of the malady was immediately succeeded by three months of depression and horrible delusion. These 3 cases, however, and the exceptional case (XIII), terminated very suddenly in convulsed coma or apoplexy long before the disease had run out to its natural conclusion in exhaustion, before the cycle of organic change was completed, or indeed before it was yet in mid-career; while in the 2 instances which terminated in exhaustion, and in which the right thalamus was the smaller, melancholic mania and delusions decidedly predominated. In the 2 remaining alternating cases the thalami were equally atrophied or softened.

It is remarkable that, of the 19 instances of unsymmetrical thalami, in 14 change of dimension in the right ganglion produced the disparity. This, on the supposition that the right thalamus is that of emotional pain, is exactly what the history of the malady would lead us to expect. Painful moral shocks, to which general paralysis is, in the great majority of known histories, indubitably traceable, had, at the outset of the disease, initiated in the right thalamus that passive hyperæmia which, if the case last long enough, ends in atrophy, softening, or degeneracy.

The structures adjacent to the thalami are those which, next to themselves, are the most commonly and most seriously implicated. These adjacent organs are not only near, but continuous with, the thalami. They are the commissura mollis, the four-pillared longitudinal fornix, the crura cerebri, and the floor of the third ventricle.

The soft commissure is not to be regarded as a separate cerebral structure, but as an integral part of the thalamic apparatus. Composed principally of gray matter, it partakes more of the nature of a ganglion than of a commissure, and any lesion of it presupposes a profounder lesion of the thalami themselves. Often wanting, or most recognisably damaged, when the thalami are merely softened or atrophied, its destruction or more conspicuous lesion is simply owing to its tenuity, and is mainly due to the solvent properties of the serum, which, natural to all the ventricles, gravitates when in increased quantity into the cleft of the third.

Of 26 cases, in 12 the commissura mollis was wanting or broken down; in 11 not a vestige of it remained, while in the 1 remaining case a few shreds of it hung from the less implicated ganglion. In 6 cases it was markedly softened, in a condition prepared for solution by the ventricular serum. In 5 instances it was healthy or indurated, and in 3 its state was not recorded. In 2 (VI and VIII) of the cases in which the commissure is registered as healthy, it would have been probably more correct to have described as not softened; it was, in truth, harder and darker than usual, and in a condition analogous to that of the contiguous thalami. It shared their degeneracy.

It may be generally stated that in all long and acute cases the soft commissure is wanting, broken down, or on the verge of diffluence.

The *fornix* was found to be markedly changed in 22 out of 26 cases; of these, in 10 instances it was dif-

fluent, in 6 extremely soft, and in 6 small and degenerated. Of the 4 remaining cases, in 3 it was healthy,
and in 1 its condition was not recorded. The most
usual sites of softening of the fornix are its anterior pillars, its body, and the vertical fibres which connect it
with the lower surface of the corpus callosum. The
streaming fibres of the posterior and inferior ventricular
cornua are rarely or never diffluent, or even softened.
In extreme cases, as in Case XI, the whole body and
anterior pillars are quite diffluent, and, the velum interpositum being broken down, lie, an amorphous and
irrecognisable mass, deep in the cleft of the third ventricle. In Case XIV a very similar but less marked
condition obtained. As, in this instance, the velum interpositum was entire, the complete disintegration of the
fornix was hardly possible. The thalami in both cases
were markedly softened, and, as specimens of paralytic
mania and melancholia, it would be difficult to over-
state their respective intensity, or the extravagance of
their peculiar delusions. The more usual locations of
diffluence, however, are the anterior pillars and the callo-
fornal fibres. In attempting to retrovert the corpus
callosum and fornix, the vertical fibres connecting them
are found to be diffluent, so that the two commissures
cannot be turned back together. The upper aspect of
the fornix falls, as it were, from the soffit of the corpus
callosum, which has the appearance of health. Coincident with this diffluence of the callo-fornal fibres, the
body of the commissure is, in most cases, similarly
affected, and is always softened; so that it cannot be
turned back entire from the velum interpositum, but has
usually to be scraped off, or detached in shreds from
that membrane. Occasionally only half of the body of

the fornix is diffluent or softened, the morbid process stopping abruptly at the raphé. The diffluence of the anterior pillars rarely pervades their entirety, though always their circumference. Flocculent externally, and its contour no longer perfect, the disruption of the whole pillar is seldom complete. It sometimes happens that the tissues about the insertion of the pillars of the fornix into the thalami are the only diffluent parts of the commissure. Diffluence of the fornix nearly always bears a direct proportion to a similar thalamic condition, and is constantly associated with intense psychical symptoms.

Softening of the fornix without diffluence is, of course, merely the previous phase of the latter condition. When the malady does not run on to its natural termination of exhaustion, and the patient is cut off by some intercurrent malady, the fornix is found softened, but still completely retaining its complicated outline. If the patient had lived, the softening would doubtless soon have merged into diffluence. In the less marked cases, whether of the elated or melancholic variety, the fornix is, not seldom, merely softened. Fornical softening has the same habitats as diffluence of the commissure, namely, the callo-fornal fibres, the body, and anterior pillars.

In 4 instances the fornix was degenerated, and in 2 atrophied, without apparent pravity of tissue. In the former cases, the callo-fornal fibres presented a very singular appearance. These fibres, no longer white, opaque, and of the usual cerebral tenacity, were of a dirty-buff colour, of horny diaphaneity, and very tough and ductile. In Case VIII this condition was true of the whole longitudinal commissure, which was, moreover, studded by sudamina-like elevations. In Cases IX, XXI, and XXIII, this peculiar corneous degeneration was strictly confined to the callo-fornal fibres. In Cases VI and XXVI, the fornix, though very small, was otherwise healthy; it was in a condition of simple atrophy. In 3 cases the longitudinal commissure is described as healthy. Whether the fornix deserved, in these instances, that compendious appellation, is perhaps doubtful; for, though there was no apparent structural change, it was smaller, though not markedly so, than the healthy commissure usually is. The quasi-healthy fornices of general paralysis, when compared with those of other mental maladies, are evidently of diminished volume; they are, probably, in an early stage of atrophy, uncomplicated by degeneration.

The mental symptoms of the three cases in which the fornix is recorded as healthy, were far below the average of paralytic intensity.

The septum lucidum and corpora albicantia are appendages of the fornix. They accordingly often participate in its lesion. The two laminæ of the septum lucidum are, however, less frequently implicated to the same extent as the body, the anterior pillars, or callofornal fibres of the longitudinal commissure. Only in a solitary and very intense case was the partition between the corpora striata broken down. More usually it is softened, so that, by the diminution of its cohesion, it is no longer able to retain its smooth, unwrinkled appearance, but, its height being at the same time greatly abridged, it is arranged in a series of bulgings with intervening depressions. But the commonest condition of the septum lucidum is that of mere diminution of volume, without change of structure—of simple atrophy, in short. It sometimes happens that the blood-vessels on one side of the septum are numerous, bright, and ramifying, while on the other side they are entirely wanting, or few, pale, and unbranched. When this latter condition obtains, the same peculiarities are equally observable on the surfaces of the corpus striatum, and of the thalamus of the same side. They are always an index to the solely or more affected thalamus.

The corpora albicantia are mere twists in the fornix, and, like its posterior pillars, are composed of delicately thin but compact medullary fibres covering gray matter. They are more frequently and more manifestly implicated in the damage of the fornix than the septum lucidum, a condition of things for which their closer connexion with the thalami would naturally prepare us. Of 26 cases, in 7 instances one or both corpora albicantia were diffluent, in 5 softened, in 8 small but otherwise healthy, in 2 normal, and in 4 their condition was not recorded. The diffluence of these bodies is of very varying degree and extent. In the most intense cases of paralytic mania or melancholia, it not unfrequently happens that only one corpus albicans is recognisable: sometimes there is no trace of the other; more usually a small, ragged, brownish mass occupies the place, and is the only vestige of the softened and nearly dissolved body. This absence or disorganization is nearly always on the same side as the more or only softened thalamus. Softening of these bodies, however, does not always go this length. The ganglia are often clearly marked by their mass, but not by their form or colour. They no longer deserve to be described as albicantia, and hardly as mammillaria. Of a dirty-brown colour, flocculent, flattened and expanded, they present a complete contrast to the pure-white, well-defined prominence natural to them. These peculiarities are clearly owing to the diffluence and solution of their thin, external white coating, and to the consequent exposure and softening of the subjacent gray matter. This condition is often only observable in one corpus. In mere softening of the corpora albicantia they retain their white colour, the lesion not having attained the enclosed gray matter. They nevertheless are seldom round or naturally prominent, but expanded, flattened, and not distinct in contour. Comparative atrophy of these bodies is to be presumed when, though healthy in appearance and consistence, they are unusually small. This condition was observed in 8 instances.

The floor of the third ventricle, behind the optic commissure, including the tuber cinereum and substantia perforata, is often deeply implicated in the discoverable lesions of general paralysis. Of 26 cases, in 7 the gray tuber was diffluent and ruptured, in 8 thin and soft, in 7 healthy, and in 4 its condition was not recorded. The first instances of ruptured tuber cinereum, which occurred to me, I regarded as accidental and rare cadaveric appearances. Instances of this peculiar lesion, however, so increased, and were found so usually after certain marked cerebral symptoms, while, with the absence of these symptoms, the tuber was entire, that my notion of its cadaveric origin gave way, and was replaced by the conviction that, so far from being a post-mortem lesion, and therefore unimportant, it was one which immediately preceded, and was, in fact, the potential cause of those marked cerebral symptoms which invariably ended in speedy death. In nearly every case in which the tuber cinereum has been found ruptured, death has been immediately preceded by unconvulsed coma of some hours' duration. The patients, indeed, exhausted and worn down to skin and bone by the intensity of their mental symptoms, had hung on the verge of existence for days or weeks, when profound coma has supervened, and in a few hours terminated fatally. In Case XVIII the convulsions of which the patient had been the subject for several weeks had all but disappeared, when, a few hours before death, he became motionless and comatose. Diffluence of the tuber rarely occurs but in the most intense cases. The consequences of the lesion are clear enough. The third ventricle, no longer having a floor composed of cerebral tissue, has no longer one capable of retaining the serum, the effusion of which is natural to the ventricles. Its cleft is now only separated by the pia mater from the subarachnoid space. Even should this slender flooring remain intact, its facility for transudation is manifest. The ventricular serum in fact, if the pia mater be intact, traverses that membrane by endosmosis, and, if ruptured, flows through the hole in it into the subarachnoid space. The rupture of the tuber cinereum is all the more fatal, as it probably usually happens that the actual cause of the rupture of the softened or semi-diffluent body is an accumulation of serum in the ventricles. The weight of this fluid in the most depending part of the brain brings the additional and, as it would seem, irresistible agency of gravity to bear upon the tuber, already on the point of giving way. The *sudden* accession of this large quantity of serum into the subarachnoid space (itself probably already containing an abnormal quantity of the fluid natural to it) is the immediate cause of the supervention of unconvulsed coma. What had before the rupture been a centrifugal pressure on the whole encephalon, acting from the centre towards the circumference, is by the rupture converted into a centripetal pressure, acting from the whole surface of the brain on its central organs. Of the respective dangers of these two compressions there is, I think, little doubt. In chronic hydrocephalus, the whole ventricular cavity is immensely distended by serum with no remarkable cerebral disturbance, certainly often without coma or convulsions. The gradual effusion of the fluid is probably the principal cause of its comparative harmlessness, to which, however, its site not a little contributes. There is little doubt that the attacks of epileptiform convulsions, and the evanescent coma or hemiplegia, to which general paralytics are so subject, are owing to the *sudden* effusion of a small quantity of serum into the ventricles, while the fatal profound coma of the malady is the result of the sudden effusion of a large quantity of serum into the subarachnoid space. The greater peril of subarachnoid or peripheral over intraventricular or central effusion is not difficult to explain. That an effusion may be exclusively subarachnoid or intraventricular, ordinary post-mortem examinations abundantly prove; though the conjunction of the two conditions is, on the other hand, only too common. Now, it is clear that the cerebral condition (whatever it may be) which produces intraventricular effusion, must be incomparably less in extent and intensity than that which results in copious subarachnoid effusion. The small extent of the whole ventricular cleft, when compared with the immense area of the subarachnoid space, following as it does the windings of every convolution, and penetrating

to the bottom of the spinal canal, demonstrates at once
the total imparity (as far as imminence of danger is con-
cerned) of effusion into the ventricles and beneath the
arachnoid. The membranes, whence alone the ventricular serum can be effused, are that lining the ventricles,
the choroid plexuses, and velum interpositum, while the
source of the subarachnoid serum is the immense layer
of pia mater from the vertex to the coccyx. It is probable that the whole pia mater participates, though certainly not quite equally, in the cause, whatever it may be,
of subarachnoid serous effusion; that this is so can
scarcely be doubted, from the fact that, in all instances
of copious cephalic subarachnoid effusion, the outpour
from the spinal canal, on slight dependence of the head, is
immense. A mere comparison of the extent of the affected
surfaces in ventricular and subarachnoid effusion is, therefore, a sufficient warrant for the assertion of the greater
peril of the latter condition. But the direction of the
pressure is perhaps quite as important an element in the
superior peril of subarachnoid effusion as the extent of the
membrane affected. If serum be suddenly effused into
the ventricles, the amount of the subarachnoid serum remaining the same, the pressure, acting at first only on
the walls or contents of the ventricles, is rapidly propa-
gated to the encephalic periphery, where, meeting with
the natural subarachnoid serum, the pressure is at once
diffused by it over the whole myolencephalic circumference. Thus the small amount of pressure, of which the
ventricular serum is capable, is rendered comparatively
innocuous by its diffusion over a very large surface.
Such a pressure is no doubt potent to produce convulsions, semi-coma, stupor, or evanescent hemiplegia, but
impotent for the causation of profound or fatal coma.

The sudden effusion of subarachnoid serum, on the contrary, while it is a symptom of a far more extended, and probably more severe morbid condition, is from its position and mechanical action a phenomenon in the highest degree fraught with peril. As I have before mentioned, it is probable that the whole congested pia mater simultaneously exudes serum, though, from its natural slighter vascularity on the pons, medulla oblongata, and spinal cord, certainly not with equal copiousness. If this be so, supposing the intraventricular serum to remain the same, the whole concentric pressure of the encephalic periphery is directed towards the point of least resistance or fulness, namely, the central or ventricular region of the cerebrum ; while, on the other hand, supposing the plexus choroides and velum interpositum to be similarly affected with the rest of the pia mater, and to exude serum into the ventricles at the same time and rate, the whole brain will be evidently compressed at once from its centre and circumference. In the former condition, the compression from the whole cerebral circumference towards the centre would at once produce profound coma; while in the latter, life would appear hardly for a moment compatible with a cerebral pressure at once eccentric and concentric. Midway between these two conditions is the state, as regards pressure, of the paralytic encephalon when the tuber cinereum is ruptured. Supposing the subarachnoid serum to be at the moment of rupture of normal quantity (which perhaps is not very likely), it is at once augmented by the sudden accession of the intraventricular serum flowing into it through the ruptured tuber; a morbid increase which goes on steadily advancing by the continuous flow of freshly secreted intraventricular serum. Though by the rupture the possibility of centrifugal pressure is for ever terminated, it at once initiates a condition of things, which, commencing in slight and sudden centripetal compression, soon ends, by the gradual draining away of the intraventricular serum into the subarachnoid space and by its accumulation there, in irretrievable converging cerebral compression and death, after some hours of motionless coma, sometimes with difficulty distinguishable from death.

The crura cerebri.—Of 26 cases, in 2 (VII and XVI) the crura cerebri were diffluent, in 11 softened or flattened, in 7 healthy, and in 6 their condition was not recorded. The more implicated crus will be usually found to correspond in side with the more affected thalamus. Sometimes, as indeed in both cases of their diffluence, the crura cerebri are more changed than the thalami. In Case VII, the thalami being only slightly atrophied, the crura cerebri were internally softened to diffluence; and in Case XVI, while the thalami were only softened externally, the whole right crus was diffluent. In the 10 cases (IV, XI, XIV, XV, XVII, XIX, XX, XXIV, XXV, XXVI) of softened but not diffluent crura cerebri, there was in nearly each instance a certain correspondence between the thalamic and the cerebro-crural lesions. When both thalami were softened equally, so were both crura; when both thalami were affected, but not equally, the same difference obtained between the changed crura; and where only one thalamus, only one crus was affected. This latter conjunction was remarkably conspicuous in Case XV, in which the left thalamus and the left crus cerebri were proportionably diminished in size. In Case XXI, coincident with diminution of the right thalamus, the corresponding crus cerebri was flattened, but not soft.

The great exceptions to the ventricular lesions of

general paralysis, whether as regards the walls or the contents of the clefts, are the corpus callosum and corpora striata. It is true that the condition of these important bodies in some instances deviates from health, but never widely. While the adjacent organs present very conspicuous lesions, the great transverse commissure and anterior cerebral ganglia are either healthy or very insignificantly changed. Diffluence, or even marked softening of these bodies, is, in general paralysis, quite unknown, their most appreciable lesion being a trifling and superficial diminution of coherence.

In 16 instances the *corpus callosum* was quite healthy, in 2 its condition was not recorded, and in 8 it was very slightly softened.

The *corpora striata*, rarely altered in consistence, do not always retain their symmetry. When *there is* a difference in size between the two great anterior cerebral ganglia, the abnormal ganglion is always, or nearly always, on the same side as the unsymmetrical thalamus. In 11 cases, in which one thalamus was the smaller, so likewise was the corpus striatum of the same side: in 1 case the right thalamus and right corpus striatum were the larger, though not commensurately so; and in 1 instance these ganglia of the right side were equally bloodless and channelled, that being the sole discoverable deviation from health, among the central ganglia. In 1 instance, the atrophy of the great central ganglia was on different sides. In but 1 instance was the corpus striatum exclusively affected, and then only slightly; in 2 instances (Cases XIV and XVI) the surfaces of both corpora striata were softened, a more extended and deeper softening existing in the adjacent thalami. In 2 cases the surface of the striated bodies was not round, but undulated. The interior of these organs I never recollect to have seen disorganized, conglomerated, or softened.

When speaking of ruptured tuber cinereum, I stated my belief that, to trifling and exclusive intraventricular effusion, are due the sudden but easily remediable epileptiform seizures of general paralysis; while to converging subarachnoid, or to it and intraventricular serous effusion combined, is due the profound motionless or convulsed fatal coma. The flitting hemiplegic attacks, with or without convulsion of the affected side, I entirely attribute to the sudden effusion of serum exclusively in one or other lateral ventricle. This *limitation* of effusion is only possible on the supposition that it is confined to one posterior or to one inferior ventricular cornu; for the want of communication between these cavities on opposite sides (except by the opening common to them and the anterior cornua, the foramen of Monro), is the only explanation of the means by which a free aqueous fluid can be confined to one ventricle.

The inferior ventricular horn presents nearly every facility for the retention of fluid; while from its position adjacent to the crura cerebri, and from the many important structures with which it comes in contact in its winding course, distension would seem to render its compressed walls peculiarly liable to affect many and distant parts of the nervous and muscular systems. The retentive power of the cornua ammonis would be indubitable even without the presence of the choroid plexuses, which, acting as sponges, while they prevent or reduce to their minima the effects of the pressure, ensure the retention of the serum for a given time at least in the inferior ventricular cornua. That the choroid plexus contributes to the retention of serum in the descending horn of the lateral ventricle is certain, from the œdematous condition in which it is often found after death, and from the presence of the large vesicles or bullæ with which it is so frequently found studded: in a word, these convoluted folds of pia mater are eminently hygrometric. This absorbent power has probably been conferred on it to prevent the accumulation of a large amount of serum in the lowermost parts of the inferior ventricular horn, where, from the immediate proximity of the crus cerebri, its presence would be in the highest degree prejudicial. It is precisely to the accumulation of serum in, or to its sudden effusion into, the lowermost bend of the inferior ventricular horn, where it is out of reach of the absorbent choroid, that the evanescent hemiplegia, coma, or convulsions of general paralysis are reasonably attributable. The remote or essential cause of the effusion and seizures is no doubt thalamic disorganization, atrophy, or pravity, the accidental or immediate cause probably being the accumulation of hardened fæces in the large intestines, or the chilling of the whole cutaneous surface by a sudden accession of severe atmospheric cold. Whatever may be the immediately preceding cause of the serous effusion, it occurs in the close vicinity of the structures, the lesions of which so obviously assert themselves as the essential causes. If the effusion take place in both inferior cornua, the paralysis is universal; while, if it be limited to one, hemiplegia of the opposite side ensues. At the first discovery of the seizure, it usually happens that the hemiplegia is not as yet established, universal paralysis obtaining. After a brisk enema and the evacuation of a copious scybalous stool, hemiplegia is, by the recovery of one side, developed. The serum has been absorbed from the less distended inferior cornu.

In the more affected cornu, its sudden distension is greatly mitigated by the absorption of the serum, as far as possible, by the choroid plexus, but the lowermost part of the cornu not being attained by that fold of pia mater, it is still distended and compressed by the fluid. The actual cause of the hemiplegia would appear to be pressure on the adjacent crus cerebri. Aided by purgatives, and possibly by the recumbent posture, which perhaps brings the fluid within reach of the absorbent choroid, the trifling dregs of serum are removed; and the *vis medicatrix naturæ* soon restores to the now no longer compressed crus cerebri the dynamic status it possessed before the seizure. It will be usually found that the hemiplegia is on the side opposite to the more affected thalamus; this, however, is by no means a constant occurrence. Of several consecutive transient hemiplegic attacks, it likewise usually happens that they occur on the same side; but there are exceptions to this rule.

This appears to me the only reasonable explanation of the fugitive hemiplegic seizures, with or without convulsion, which are so characteristic of our malady; seizures commencing quite suddenly, and at first emulating the importance of apoplexy; then developing by their half-cure hemiplegia, which, in its turn, under the simplest possible treatment, vanishes in a few hours, or, at most, days, leaving behind it not a trace of symptoms so remarkable and, at first sight, so tremendous.

CHAPTER VII.

TREATMENT.

THE treatment of general paralysis is a subject which I approach reluctantly, and not without a feeling of despondence. The manifest hopelessness of the majority of cases, which have come under my notice, has induced me to regard the disease rather from a physiological than a therapeutic point of view; rather as a rich and unexplored mine of physico-psychical curiosities than as a curable malady. As, however, our knowledge increases, it will be probably found not more incurable than phthisis, albuminuria, or valvular disease of the heart; that is, though still incurable, largely palliable.

The first stage of the malady, that which precedes insanity, is indeed hopeful; though perhaps from our comparative ignorance of its symptoms, we may permit ourselves to be unphilosophically sanguine of its curability.

To calm the fury of paralytic exaltation, to raise paralytic melancholy from its depression, and to liberate its subject from an asylum, is something; but it is merely to add an useless member to a population already large enough, to restore to the world a man able indeed to enjoy, but not to utilise his freedom. General paralysis, therefore, has this disadvantage compared with other incurable chronic diseases, that while the palliation of these often adds to the floating capital of energy and talent, by raising from their beds of sickness persons useful or distinguished in their generation, men who, though physically feeble, yet stimulated by ambition or affection, often "put' to shame the puny efforts" of the more robust,—its palliation restores to society, what society can well do without, semi-demented, elated, or depressed persons. To a part, and not the least important of what I have to say on this subject, allusion has been already incidentally made (see p. 52).

Nearly the whole treatment of general paralysis consists in the mitigation of symptoms; and to calm intense paralytic excitement by Hyoscyamus, and to support by a generous but unstimulating diet a body exhausted by sleeplessness, by frightful or exalted fancies, constitutes nearly the whole of the palliative treatment.

Henbane is a remedy of which the paralytic maniac seems peculiarly and largely tolerant. Given in sufficient doses it rarely fails to diminish, if not to check, intense excitement. When the patient is not very feeble, a scruple of the extract is not too large a dose to begin with. This may be repeated twice or thrice a day if the maniacal symptoms be not mitigated by the first dose. If after the first diminution or abeyance of the maniacal symptoms they should return with equal or increasing violence, apparently from the nervous system getting accustomed to the drug, the dose may be increased by five or ten grains as often as the effect of the previous dose appears to have worn off. On this plan I have constantly given half a drachm, frequently two scruples, and more than once fifty grains of the extract of Hyoscyamus thrice a day. When the patient is very feeble, the dose of the extract has usually been ten grains at the commencement, and has rarely been increased beyond half a drachm.

In the medical treatment of paralytic mania, and indeed of insanity generally, it is easy enough to prescribe remedies, but often not quite so easy to induce the patient to take them; when, however, the paralytic can be induced to take the sedative regularly, it has rarely happened that the maniacal symptoms have not been checked or greatly mitigated. Sometimes, from grand or depressed fancies, from the idea that his state is above or beyond the reach of medicine, that he is so exalted or so healthy a being that medicine is either insulting or superfluous to him, or that his hopeless case renders its exhibition vain, from the delusion of poisoning, from fancied obstruction in his gullet and intestines, from imagined absence of stomach, or in the hope of death by starvation, he obstinately refuses food and physic. Sometimes he will take food but not physic, at other times physic and not food. When he refuses medicine it should be mixed with his liquid food. Porter or coffee will be found a good vehicle for henbane. When food only is refused, liquid nutriment, disguised as a drug, should be offered him from a medicine bottle. These useful deceptions are only requisite during the height of the paroxysm; as the sedative acts, a faint glimmer of returning reason usually renders their employment no longer possible or necessary. During the continuance of the most intense symptoms it will be usually found that liquid food is the only nutriment the paralytic maniac can be persuaded to take. Milk, eggs and brandy, or eggs and porter, are useful and grateful modes of administering nourishment. As what is requisite is not to stimulate but simply to sus-

tain the patient, while in this condition, four ounces of
brandy or a quart of porter will probably be enough for
him daily.

Other sedatives, besides henbane, I have often tried
in the treatment of general paralysis, but their effects
have not encouraged or even justified their continuance.
Conium, Liq. Opii sedat., morphia, the various prepara-
tions of crude opium, the aqueous and alcoholic extracts
of Cannabis indica, have, as far as my experience
goes, but little efficacy in tranquillizing the paralytic
maniac, even when given in doses unusually large.
Opium indeed is peculiarly noxious to him. It
does not tranquillize him in the least. He remains
sleepless and restless, though his contracted pupils
tell how completely he is narcotized. Stupified but
not calmed, he tumbles about his padded room in
a sort of drunken reverie. Hyoscyamus, on the other
hand, though it does not always produce sleep, rarely
fails to tranquillize, and in a most signal manner, the
patient. In half an hour after the exhibition of a scruple
or half a drachm of the extract, the paralytic raving is
at an end, though excitement, the consequence of delusion, may remain. Often, however, sound refreshing
sleep is the nearly immediate result of an adequate dose.
At the end of four or five hours the patient wakes up
quite a new person. He is now tractable and calm;
he, however, rarely remains so long, unless he be kept
under the influence of the drug. As the system gets
habituated to these large doses, it must be increased, for
if the intense symptoms be not checked the patient
speedily dies from exhaustion. The effect of Hyoscyamus is very conspicuous in those cases of paralytic
mania in which the pupils are firmly contracted. These

persons arc usually not very feeble, though their maniacal symptoms are often intense. It was in a case of this kind that the dose was gradually increased until the patient took 150 grains in the course of the day. This he not only tolerated with impunity, but took with the greatest conceivable benefit to himself and to the comfort of those about him. On its remission all his maniacal symptoms returned, on its re-exhibition they were all again mitigated; and coincident with its continued administration they all gradually faded away. The effect of Hyoscyamus in dilating the pupil is very different in different paralytics; though, when the dose is sufficiently large, every iris, whatever may have been its previous condition, is more or less signally dilated by it. Thus contracted and nearly insensible pupils dilate only slightly under the influence of henbane, while pupils of normal size and contractility are dilated wide. The dilatation of the pupil, though curious, is of little value as a therapeutic indication. Despite a largely dilated pupil, the drug must be fearlessly persevered in, and, if necessary, in increasing doses, until sleep is obtained.

The treatment of general paralysis by Hyoscyamus is not a mere ingenious device for keeping the patient quiet; it does something more than stupify him. It husbands his feeble stamina; and if, by calming him, it contributes to the comfort of his neighbours, it likewise, and by the same process, saves for the time being his own life. In this it differs patently from tartar emetic. The treatment of mania by the potassio-tartrate of antimony is nothing but a dodge, an artifice for silencing the patient by nauseating him. Its exhibition is wholly inadmissible when the patient is feeble, as all general paralytics are, or when there is any tendency to refusal of food. The maniac can only be kept quiet by being kept nauseated. When I reflect on the feeble pulse of the maniac, and on his livid cold hand, I am the more convinced of the unphilosophical, not to say the unjustifiable nature of the nauseating treatment. The coincidence of languid circulation and of intense mania is so frequent as to have impressed me with the idea that they hold the relation to each other of cause and effect; and I as much differ from those psychologists who, in the present day, attribute to mere cerebral irritation the phenomena of mania, as from those who formerly ascribed them to inflammation. A *passive* congestion of the cerebral tissues, rarely or never leading to the usual results of inflammation, is sufficiently explanatory of all maniacal symptoms. The efficacy of the sedative treatment in mania, and the total failure of the antiphlogistic plan, prove conclusively the absence of active cerebral inflammation; while the admirable results of a combination of stimulants and sedatives seem to show that all that is requisite is, by increasing the action of the heart, to relieve the cerebral congestion, the effect of a languid blood-current. An ounce of brandy or a pint of porter with half a drachm of extract of Hyoscyamus in it, will do more for the tranquillization of the patient than any number of leeches or blisters, or any amount of tartar emetic. The principal dangers to be anticipated in mania are two, namely, death by exhaustion, and coma. The only method of obviating the first of these is, to calm without lowering the patient; the same bold measures which in delirium tremens are so successful, may with some modifications, and sometimes with other drugs, be imitated in the treatment of mania. The only means of preventing the maniac's death by coma is, by increasing the rapidity and force of the cerebral blood-stream, to diminish to its minimum the chance of serous effusion. The last assertion I do not make unadvisedly ; for in all cases of partial or complete coma, with or without convulsion, happening in the course of acute, chronic, or paralytic mania, I have invariably found a more or less copious serum in the subarachnoid space or in the ventricles; and the profundity of the coma has been in direct proportion to the amount of serum effused. The cause of the effusion is only too evident. From feebleness of the heart's action, and often from a diminished elasticity of the cerebral arteries, ensues a comparative stasis of the blood in the capillaries of the brain and pia mater. The passively congested vessels relieving themselves, as elsewhere, by serous effu-sion, sudden cerebral compression and its result, coma, ensue. If this be true, the treatment of mania by so de-pressing a remedy as tartar emetic would seem incom-prehensible. The attempt to diminish intense excitement, itself the consequence of languid circulation, by depress-ing still more, and for a long time, the heart's action, is carrying out the ridiculous dogma of " Similia similibus curantur " to its extreme, its most absurd, and its most mischievous length.

Despite my low opinion of the antimonial treatment in the usual cases of mania, I have occasionally seen it justifiably employed. In instances of recurrent mania occurring in the young and robust, it has sometimes, by nauseating, tranquillized the patient. In these cases the maniac's strong physical condition is a sufficient guarantee against any danger resulting from continued nausea, and, if anorexia ensue, the robust patient can for a short time bear abstinence. Yet in these cases I do not delude myself into the idea that I am treating mania; no, I am merely quieting a noisy patient by nauseating him. By a stratagem sufficiently clumsy, by an expedient justifiable only because the patient can just tolerate it, or at most because he is not much harmed by it, I for the time being tranquillize him. But the calm does not hasten his recovery, for it is but transient. With the nausea entirely disappears the welcome lull of the maniacal symptoms.

One of the great sources of fallacy in the treatment of paralytic mania is the state of the pulse. In a large number of general paralytics, at least in half, the pulse is full, often very full, and compressible with difficulty. This, it is not improbable, has been often mistaken for the pulse of power, for an indication justifying or even imperatively calling for what is called active treatment; for venesection, for the imposition of leeches and blisters, for the application of the cupping-glasses, for the liberal exhibition of antimony, calomel, and croton oil. But this full pulse is not the result of powerful ventricular contraction; it is simply the consequence of the pulse-wave traversing an unusually good conductor of undulations, and conveying to the finger an abnormally distinct tactual impression. And what is this unusually good conductor of vibrations? The rigid arterial tube. The radial and brachial in this disease are frequently rigid and tortuous, though rarely or never ossified. Just above the bend of the elbow, or at the wrist, these arteries may be seen conspicuously pulsating. The vessels have from this circumstance the appearance of being unusually superficial; they often really are so. When the patient is emaciated, these tortuous, rigid, and superficial tubes are so manifest as to warn the practitioner of the cause of the full, hard pulse. When, however, the paralytic maniac is well covered, the full pulse, though less remarkable, is still full and hard enough to mislead the medical attendant. The latter, comparing the pulse with the apparently good physical condition and with the intense maniacal excitement of the patient, imagines he has to deal with an acute cerebral disease. He opens a vein, and unintentionally bleeds palliable incipient general paralysis into immitigable maniacal dementia.

If my views regarding the immediate cause of mania be correct, its treatment by purgation has not even the doubtful merit of plausibility. On the old notion of cerebral inflammation, and in accordance with that most singular of all terms in the nosology, phrenitis (inflammation of the mind), the treatment of insanity generally by purgative drugs, however prejudicial to the patient, was at least not unphilosophical in the physician, for it was consistent with a prevailing nosopsychology. There is no necessity for determining from the head in the treatment of paralytic mania; or at least if such necessity exist, the usual means of relieving cephalic congestion must not be adopted. The proposal, therefore, to relieve a passive congestion of the head by hypercatharsis, to depress by purgatives a circulation already at a very low ebb, appears to me so manifestly unreasonable as to carry with it its own refutation. There is, moreover, a most conclusive proof of the futility of drastic purgatives in paralytic mania. One of the most usual complications of the malady is an obstinate diarrhœa, which, so far from curing the paralytic or mending his condition, speedily, if not arrested, brings the case to a fatal conclusion.

The objections I have urged against purgatives do not apply to laxatives. However averse to attempting revulsion from the head by serous evacuations from the intestines, to trying to relieve a passive oppression of the cerebral by acting on the portal circulation, I know of no more important part of the treatment of general paralysis than a rigid attention to the regularity of the bowels, than measures taken to prevent any fæcal accumulation. The presence of scybala in the intestinal tube is by far the most frequent, is indeed the only traceable cause of the convulsed seizures peculiar to general paralysis. This opinion is founded on the remarkable effect of saline enemata in the treatment of these attacks. A salt injection, in nine cases out of ten, brings away from the comatose hemiplegic an immense number of small, hard, feculent lumps. Immediately on their discharge the patient improves, the coma is less profound ; in a few hours speech returns, and in a day or two slight voluntary motions of the paralyzed limbs. No serous alvine evacuations are requisite to diminish the serous cerebral compression, but simply the removal of that condition, which is doubtless the eccentric cause of these peculiar fits, a loaded intestinal tube. As a precaution, therefore, against the most to be dreaded, but, as it would seem, most evitable complication of the malady, the bowels should be kept rigidly but gently open ; and if nature fail, measures should be taken to imitate her actions as nearly as possible. To ensure this necessary imitation the simplest and mildest laxatives are alone admissible. The Pilula Aloes c. Sapone, the Pil. Aloes c. Myrrha, the compound decoction of aloes, infusion of rhubarb, castor oil, the compound rhubarb pill, sulphur, guiacum, or brown bread, will be found sufficient for the ordinary run of paralytics. Occasionally the necessity arises for more active remedies. The coincidence of a hard, tumid abdomen, of obstinate constipation, and intense paralytic mania is not unfrequent. If for the relief of this condition the laxatives above mentioned are insufficient, if the patient be so violent as to render the administration of an enema difficult or dangerous, or if refusal of bulky physic be a prominent symptom, a drop of croton oil may be placed on the tongue, or dropped into his tea. This rarely fails to ease the loaded canal and to relieve the maniacal symptoms. Injections can now, if necessary, be given; or if the disinclination to take medicine have passed away, mild purgatives will be readily swallowed. An account of the procedure to be adopted immediately on the discovery of a paralytic seizure will be found at page 52.

Hitherto, in my remarks on the treatment of general paralysis, no mention has been made of any remedial scheme for the arrest of that organic change in the central region of the encephalon, to which all the physico-psychical symptoms of the malady are to be traced. I have contented myself with describing the means by which the intensity of paralytic mania may be lessened, and with pointing out those so-called remedies which, in its treatment, are to be especially avoided. It remains for me to glance at a plan of radical treatment, by which has been attempted the arrest of the organic cerebral change, and, as it has been imagined by some, not without success. In those cases in which the semi-dementia is only as yet incipient, in which the memory is not greatly impaired, the delusions not extravagant, nor the excitement intense, the continued employment of small doses of mercury has appeared to stay the onward progress of the disease. The patient, after taking three or five grains of blue pill every night for two or three months, becomes calm, and the tranquillity has been permanent. But inasmuch as this mild mercurial course has been tried only in the less severe instances of the malady, and as it has repeatedly happened that similar trifling cases have become calm without any mercury at all, it is quite an open question whether the diminution or disappearance of maniacal symptoms, after the long-continued exhibition of small doses of mercury, is a post hoc or a propter hoc, a sequence or a consequence. The duty of the medical man, however, often compels him to use remedies in whose efficacy he does not implicitly trust, and the mode of whose action he cannot trace. Though doubtless we should endeavour as far as possible to obtain clear notions of the actions of remedies, it would ill become us, as disciples of, as it at present exists, the least fixed and most fallible of all sciences, to deprive our patient of any possible chance of recovery, because we may be uncertain whether the reputation of any given drug is deserved, or because its modus operandi is obscure. Swayed by these considerations, I think we should in fit cases give the general paralytic all the chance of benefit derivable from a prolonged but mild mercurial course. Some practitioners are in the habit of giving a drachm of Liq. Hydrarg. Bichloridi, equivalent to one sixteenth of a grain of the sublimate, three times a day, in the treatment of this malady. Of the result of this plan I have but slight experience, for I have seldom tried it. Its reasonableness is however so evident, that, if it cannot command, it at least deserves success. It is probable that a combination of this method with henbane might be of great value in the treatment of intense paralytic mania. A scruple or half a drachm of Ext. Hyoscyami, and a sixteenth of a grain of the bichloride of mercury, twice or thrice a day, always provided it were possible to give it regularly, would be a combination fulfilling the principal indications for treatment which the malady presents. The sublimate might act beneficially on, might perhaps arrest the incipient disorganization of the central cerebral structures; and the Hyoscyamus, by subduing the mania, would economise the patient's strength, and enable him to tolerate the mercurial with greater ease.[1]

The general paralytic, no matter what his mental condition, is greatly depressed by cold. It invariably happens that the mortality in an asylum is greater in winter than at any other season. The cause of this is

---

[1] I have, since writing the above, in about a dozen cases, tried the suggested combination of the Bichloride of Mercury and the Extract of Hyoscyamus, not, however, with any encouraging results, beyond the transient tranquillization of the patient by the sedative.

The extract has been usually given dissolved in water. This turbid draught, from its unsightly appearance, the patient has sometimes refused to take. The objection to this method of exhibiting Henbane is the presence of the inert green extractive matter, which may, however, be removed by subsidence or filtration. During the last two years, I have used with the best effect an elegant preparation which may be called "Liquor Hyoscyami." It has been prepared in the following manner: Dissolve ℥xx Ext. Hyoscy., in a sufficient quantity of boiling water, let it stand for twenty-four hours for the extractive matter to subside; then by the syphon, remove the clear supernatant liquor. Treat the precipitate again with boiling water, and, after a lapse of twenty-four hours, again remove the clear liquor; mix the liquors, and evaporate to ℥xl.

The Liquor Hyoscyami, thus obtained, is half the strength of the extract, all the therapeutic virtue of which it contains. In doses of twenty, forty, sixty, or eighty drops, it has been daily employed with the best effects, calming the patient, and dilating the pupil as readily as the inelegant solution of the extract formerly employed. It is especially convenient in cases of refusal of medicine, as, being nearly tasteless, it can be given in coffee or porter, without the patient in the least suspecting his food is drugged.

the death of general paralytics by bronchitis, diarrhœa, exhaustion, or coma. During the summer, semi-demented paralytics pass a very tolerable existence ; but, nipped by the first cold day, they rapidly succumb, unless kept constantly in a genial atmosphere, and well sustained by food and stimulants. The converse of this is sometimes observed : a paralytic, who has been, during the winter and early spring, stationary, silent, utterly demented, and dirty in his habits, becomes, as the weather gets warmer, at first less stationary; then his silence is broken by monosyllabic answers, his habits become clean, soon he remembers a name; presently he attempts, awkwardly enough, to perform some familiar act; he improves daily, until he is at length a cheerful, industrious, talkative perhaps, semi-demented man. This condition may be stationary until the cold weather again depresses him into hybernation, or it may go on increasing until it becomes a furious paroxysm of paralytic mania.

Bronchitis, of a low type, is a troublesome and often a fatal complication of general paralysis in severe weather. Unless grappled with at its outset, it rapidly assumes the aspect and the peril of suffocative pulmonitis. The patient may go to bed with an apparently trifling catarrh. In the morning he has severe dyspnœa, the surface is hot and livid, the eyeballs are congested and staring, the face and lips purple, the mucous rattle in the bronchi loud and coarse. If this condition be not relieved, and it rarely can be, the paralytic in a few hours dies semi-comatose, from the circulation of un-aerated blood in the brain and in the tissues of the heart. The explanation of the cause and of the rapid course of this peculiar bronchitis is evident enough.

Acute bronchitis, especially in its epidemic form, is never a very tractable malady. The great danger is of course slow asphyxia, from the tubes becoming choked by mucous secretion. The natural safeguard against this is frequency and vigour of respiratory effort. By a powerful inspiration air is drawn, however imperfectly and in small quantity, through the mucus to the vesicular membrane; by a powerful expiration the system is relieved of its excrementitious carbon. In paralytic bronchitis, on the other hand, these elements of safety are greatly abridged. From the feebleness of the paralytic's inspiration, the air with difficulty forces its way through the mucus-clogged tubes to the vesicular membrane; and though it reach the membrane, it reaches it in insufficient quantity. In consequence of the feeble expiration, the excreted carbonic acid cannot extricate itself from the vesicles of the lungs. This diminution of blood-aerating power, and the abeyance of the ability to expectorate, the bronchial effusion the while continuing to increase, is a condition of things only for a few hours compatible with life. The nearly complete destruction of expectorating power is no doubt mainly attributable to the advancing paralytic feebleness of the respiratory muscles, though the comparative anæsthesia of the paralytic's pulmonary mucous membrane certainly plays its part in the production of suffocative bronchitis.

It is evident, therefore, that a rational mode of treatment of paralytic bronchitis will simply be an attempt to augment the power of the respiratory effort, and to hasten the removal of the accumulated bronchial effusion. All the usual methods of treating acute bronchitis by tartar emetic and similar lowering measures are, therefore, out of the question, as, even supposing they checked the progress of the malady, the paralytic would none the less die of suffocative exhaustion, from inability to clear the bronchial tubes of their previous mucous load. The only treatment combining the two indications above mentioned, is a combination of stimulants and expectorants, with the simultaneous employment of blisters to the chest. The best stimulant that can be given is brandy and eggs; and I have seen much good resulting from the exhibition of ℨss or ℨj of the Acet. Scillæ, forty minims or a drachm of the compound Sulphuric Æther, out of camphor mixture, every four hours. This combination, and the application of a large blister between or beneath the scapulæ, are certainly followed by an evident remission of the dyspnœa; all the symptoms of impending suffocation and of the circulation of venous blood are greatly mitigated, and sometimes entirely subside. It is almost needless to add, that the patient's chamber should be kept at a uniform and genial temperature.

Diarrhœa is an occasional complication of the last stage of general paralysis. Though it is rarely the immediate cause of death, the feebleness it induces often hastens the fatal issue. Antacids, chalk, and aromatics, I have found quite inoperative against it. Dilute sulphuric acid, in half drachm doses, sometimes checks it, and sulphate of copper rarely fails to do so, if given in time and in sufficient quantity. Half a grain of the sulphate and an equal dose of powdered opium, given every four hours, will usually stay any diarrhœa that may occur in the course of general paralysis.

In consequence of the lowered organic innervation of general paralysis, and of the participation of the skin in this depression, the dirty habits of the paralytic maniac sometimes produce sores on the hips and over the sacrum, and often cause discoloration of the skin of those regions. The latter circumstance is not seldom the harbinger of the former. The only means of preventing these sometimes not very tractable complications, is keeping the patient rigidly clean, and never, if he be dirty, permitting him to lie in his urinous sheets. This plan, if it could always be fully carried out, would doubtless be always successful. But the intense excitement and violence of the paralytic maniac render it sometimes impracticable. The skin now gets discoloured; it is of a dirty-livid tint, and is evidently unhealthy. If this morbid condition be not rectified, it soon gives way. The best plan I have seen of averting this danger is by painting the unhealthy, livid, but as yet unbroken skin with a saturated solution of nitrate of silver in spirit of nitric æther. The advantages of this application are several: 1st, it dries rapidly; 2dly, it forms a thin varnish over the unhealthy skin, by which the latter is protected from the urine; 3dly, it stimulates the cuticle to throw off the unhealthy layer, and by the same stimulation ensures that the succeeding layer shall be more healthy than that it replaces. The application should be continued on the desquamation of the cuticle, if the dirty habits of the patient be not cured by that time. Towards the close of the malady, when the physico-psychical condition is at its lowest ebb, when the dementia is complete, and nearly all but organic motions are in abeyance, it is difficult to prevent the formation of sores on any part of the body which can be influenced, in however trifling a manner, by pressure. To prevent the skin of the sacrum, of the heels, the hips, or the scapulæ, giving way extensively, the water-bed or the strap-bed may be employed, though, as it will be found, not always with complete success. The water or air-cushion is likewise a useful auxiliary. The mere mutual pressure of the inner aspect of the knees sometimes produces sores on these parts. The interposition of a soft pad will sometimes avert, or retard their formation. If extensive abrasion of the skin happen, it usually occurs in fat and flabby paralytics of fair complexion. The highly ammoniacal urine of these persons rapidly acts on their skin, a tissue which, in common with all others of the paralytic's body, is now at the lowest degree of vitality compatible with life. The skin of these persons becomes discoloured by the least pressure; thus, the upper arms are often slightly ecchymosed, as the mere result of the handling necessary in changing their bed-clothes, or sustaining them erect while eating. The bruises, the consequences of these most necessary attentions, have frequently been mistaken for the marks of violence, and have been most undeservedly adduced, by those who should have known better, as the evidences of cruelty.

The treatment of paralytic sores is of the simplest kind. It may be perhaps summed up in two axioms.

First: rigid cleanliness of the paralytic is to be enjoined on the attendants. The medical attendant should see that this injunction is acted up to, a desirable consummation which he is not likely to witness without his own strict and frequent supervision.

Secondly: the avoidance of poultices, except where sloughs are to be brought away. When the paralytic's sores are, as they nearly always are at first, superficial, wet lint and oil-silk will be found quite sufficient to clean the surface. When the pellicle of slough is removed, dry lint kept on by a large piece of Emp. Plumbi, spread upon *thick* leather, will be found a useful and an effectual remedy. If the patient, with this application on his hips or over his sacrum, lie on either of these parts, the gentle pressure will prove an efficacious stimulant to the protected sores; and in many cases render unnecessary the application of chemical stimuli—the nitrate of silver, the sulphate of copper, or the nitrico-oxyde of mercury. If large sloughs form, linseed and charcoal poultices are requisite. Should the patient have vigour enough to throw off the slough, a healthy condition of the cavity usually follows. The rapidity with which large and deep paralytic sores fill up is very remarkable, a celerity of reproduction only surpassed by the still more rapid healthy healing of wounds, and of filling up of sores in epileptics.

THE END.

Classics in Psychiatry

An Arno Press Collection

American Psychiatrists Abroad. 1975

Arnold, Thomas. **Observations On The Nature, Kinds, Causes, And Prevention Of Insanity.** 1806. Two volumes in one

Austin, Thomas J. **A Practical Account Of General Paralysis, Its Mental And Physical Symptoms, Statistics, Causes, Seat, And Treatment.** 1859

Bayle, A[ntoine] L[aurent] J[esse]. **Traité Des Maladies Du Cerveau Et De Ses Membranes.** 1826

Binz, Carl. **Doctor Johann Weyer.** 1896

Blandford, G. Fielding. **Insanity And Its Treatment.** 1871

Bleuler, Eugen. **Textbook Of Psychiatry.** 1924

Braid, James. **Neurypnology.** 1843

Brierre de Boismont, A[lexandre-Jacques-François]. **Hallucinations.** 1853

Brown, Mabel Webster, compiler. **Neuropsychiatry And The War: A Bibliography With Abstracts** and **Supplement I,** October 1918. Two volumes in one

Browne, W. A. F. **What Asylums Were, Are, And Ought To Be.** 1837

Burrows, George Man. **Commentaries On The Causes, Forms, Symptoms And Treatment, Moral And Medical, Of Insanity.** 1828

Calmeil, L[ouis]-F[lorentin]. **De La Folie:** Considérée Sous Le Point De Vue Pathologique, Philosophique, Historique Et Judiciaire, Depuis La Renaissance Des Sciences En Europe Jusqu'au Dix-Neuvième Siècle. 1845. Two volumes in one

Calmeil, L[ouis] F[lorentin]. **De La Paralysie Considérée Chez Les Aliénés.** 1826

Dejerine, J[oseph Jules] and E. Gauckler. **The Psychoneuroses And Their Treatment By Psychotherapy.** [1913]

Dunbar, [Helen] Flanders. **Emotions And Bodily Changes.** 1954

Ellis, W[illiam] C[harles]. **A Treatise On The Nature, Symptoms, Causes And Treatment Of Insanity.** 1838

Emminghaus, H[ermann]. **Die Psychischen Störungen Des Kindesalters.** 1887

Esdaile, James. **Mesmerism In India,** And Its Practical Application In Surgery And Medicine. 1846

Esquirol, E[tienne]. **Des Maladies Mentales.** 1838. Three volumes in two

Feuchtersleben, Ernst [Freiherr] von. **The Principles Of Medical Psychology.** 1847

Georget, [Etienne-Jean]. **De La Folie:** Considérations Sur Cette Maladie. 1820

Haslam, John. **Observations On Madness And Melancholy.** 1809

Hill, Robert Gardiner. **Total Abolition Of Personal Restraint In The Treatment Of The Insane.** 1839

Janet, Pierre [Marie-Felix] and F. Raymond. **Les Obsessions Et La Psychasthénie.** 1903. Two volumes

Janet, Pierre [Marie-Felix]. **Psychological Healing.** 1925. Two volumes

Kempf, Edward J. Psychopathology. 1920

Kraepelin, Emil. **Manic-Depressive Insanity And Paranoia.** 1921

Kraepelin, Emil. **Psychiatrie:** Ein Lehrbuch Für Studirende Und Aerzte. 1896

Laycock, Thomas. **Mind And Brain.** 1860. Two volumes in one

Liébeault, A[mbroise]-A[uguste]. **Le Sommeil Provoqué Et Les États Analogues.** 1889

Mandeville, B[ernard] De. **A Treatise Of The Hypochondriack And Hysterick Passions.** 1711

Morel, B[enedict] A[ugustin]. **Traité Des Degénérescences Physiques, Intellectuelles Et Morales De L'Espèce Humaine.** 1857. Two volumes in one

Morison, Alexander. **The Physiognomy Of Mental Diseases.** 1843

Myerson, Abraham. **The Inheritance Of Mental Diseases.** 1925

Perfect, William. **Annals Of Insanity.** [1808]

Pinel, Ph[ilippe]. **Traité Médico-Philosophique Sur L'Aliénation Mentale.** 1809

Prince, Morton, et al. **Psychotherapeutics.** 1910

Psychiatry In Russia And Spain. 1975

Ray, I[saac]. **A Treatise On The Medical Jurisprudence Of Insanity.** 1871

Semelaigne, René. **Philippe Pinel Et Son Oeuvre Au Point De Vue De La Médecine Mentale.** 1888

Thurnam, John. **Observations And Essays On The Statistics Of Insanity.** 1845

Trotter, Thomas. **A View Of The Nervous Temperament.** 1807

Tuke, D[aniel] Hack, editor. **A Dictionary Of Psychological Medicine.** 1892. Two volumes

Wier, Jean. **Histoires, Disputes Et Discours Des Illusions Et Impostures Des Diables, Des Magiciens Infames, Sorcieres Et Empoisonneurs.** 1885. Two volumes

Winslow, Forbes. **On Obscure Diseases Of The Brain And Disorders Of The Mind.** 1860

Burdett, Henry C. **Hospitals And Asylums Of The World.** 1891-93. Five volumes. 2,740 pages on NMA standard 24x-98 page microfiche only